Breast Reduction Surgery

THE COMPLETE GUIDE TO BREAST REDUCTION SURGERY & RECOVERY

INSPIRED LIFE PRESS

First published in 2019 by Ayesha Hilton

National Library of Australia Cataloguing in Publications data:
Author: Ayesha Hilton
Title: Breast Reduction Surgery: The Complete Guide to Breast
Reduction Surgery & recovery
Subject: breast reduction surgery

Published by Inspired Life Press

Disclaimer: The material in this publication is of the nature
of general comment only and does not represent professional
advice. It is not intended to provide specific guidance for particular circumstances and should not be relied on as the basis
for any decision to take action or not take action any matters it
covers. Readers should obtain professional advice as appropriate before taking any action. To the maximum extent permitted
by law, the author and publisher disclaim all responsibility and
liability to any person, arising directly or indirectly from any
person taking or not taking action based on the information in
this book.

Medical Disclaimer: This book is not intended to provide medical advice. Please consult your doctor or surgeon for medical
information. No responsibility is taken for any medical decisions
made as a result of reading the information in this book.

Ordering Information:
Quantity sales. Special discounts are available on quantity
purchases by corporations, associations, and others. For details,
contact Ayesha Hilton at www.ayeshahilton.com

Ayesha Hilton, Breast Reduction Surgery: The Complete Guide
to Breast Reduction Surgery and Recovery. —1st ed.
ISBN eBook: 978-0-9944229-3-4 | Print: 978-0-9944229-4-1

Breast REDUCTION SURGERY

The Complete Guide to Breast
Reduction Surgery & Recovery

AYESHA HILTON

Our deepest fear is not that we are inadequate.
Our deepest fear is that we are powerful beyond measure.
It is our Light, not our Darkness, that most frightens us.

Marianne Williamson

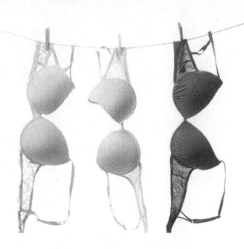

CONTENTS

PART 1: Breast Reduction Surgery

Part 2: Surgery & Recovery

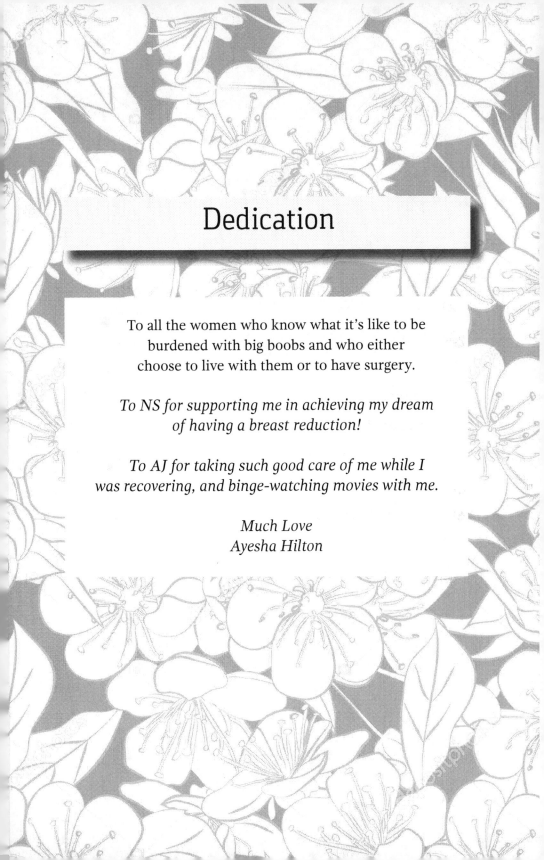

Dedication

To all the women who know what it's like to be
burdened with big boobs and who either
choose to live with them or to have surgery.

*To NS for supporting me in achieving my dream
of having a breast reduction!*

*To AJ for taking such good care of me while I
was recovering, and binge-watching movies with me.*

Much Love
Ayesha Hilton

Message from Author

Dear Reader

If you are considering having a breast reduction, let me tell you, I have been where you are now. I had been thinking of having a breast reduction for more than 20 years, but I wanted to wait until I had finished having children as I was committed to breastfeeding.

When my youngest child was two and a half, I started seriously looking into having a reduction. I found a surgeon locally, but after looking at the photos of the breast reductions in her portfolio, I wanted to find a better surgeon, and I am so thankful I did find the right surgeon for me.

After waiting so long, it is still hard for me to believe that I now have smaller breasts. My back and neck pain have been reduced as I am no longer lugging around those massive breasts.

Before I had surgery, I wrote a blog post about having a breast reduction. I was amazed by how many women contacted me. They shared with me how my story had touched them, and about their wishes to also have a reduction. Many have since gone on to have successful breast reductions themselves.

As I lay in hospital on the day of my surgery, it dawned on me that I could share my experience, and my ability to research and write, in a book to help other women considering a breast reduction. This book was born in that moment, and despite being on morphine and waking from surgery just hours before, I got out my mobile phone and began making notes.

Since then, I have spoken with many women who have had breast reduction surgery. They have shared their stories with me. Most of these women have said that having a breast reduction was the best thing they'd ever done and no regrets.

I have also connected with more women that are considering breast reduction surgery. I have listened to their questions and answered as many of them as I can in this book.

Whether you choose to have a breast reduction or not, I hope this book serves to help you make an informed decision about your body, your surgeon, and gives you insight into the recovery process. I wish I had read this book before I had surgery, as I now know so much more than I did before!

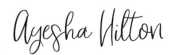

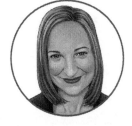

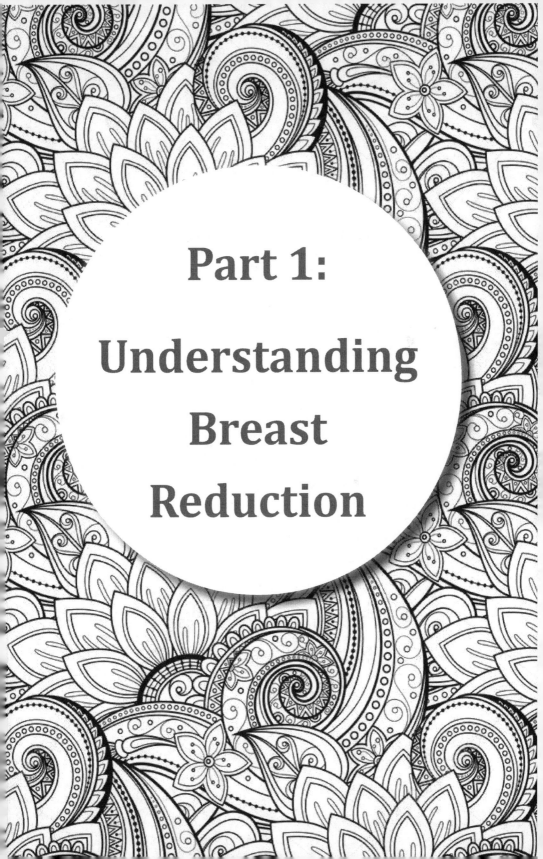

Part 1:

Understanding Breast Reduction

Part 1: Understanding Breast Reduction

Welcome to Part 1 where you will learn all about breast reduction surgery, including:

- Breast reduction techniques

- The anatomy of the breast

- The benefits and risks of breast reduction surgery

- Scarring

- Costs and insurance

- Post-op breast size

- How to find and choose a surgeon

CHAPTER 1

An Introduction to Breast Reduction

Breast Reduction, also known as **_reduction mammoplasty_**, reduces the size of your breasts and reshapes them so they are more proportionate to the rest of your body, which can greatly reduce discomfort and pain caused by large breasts.

Breast Reduction removes breast tissue, breast fat, glandular tissue and skin to make the breasts smaller, it also lifts the breast and evens out breasts of different sizes (many large busted women have one breast that is larger than the other).

To remove tissue and skin from the breast, the surgeon makes one or more cuts in the breast, removes the excess tissue and skin, and then closes with stitches.

Sometimes, the **nipple and areola** are removed and repositioned. Often the areola is resized using the "cookie cutter" method. (I used to have large areolas and now they are a normal and very round.)

Many people believe that the nipple and areola are cut off completely from your body; however, the surgeon retains blood flow to the nipple and areola so that they can be repositioned with blood flow so that they don't die off. Nipple-die-off is one of the major risks of breast reduction surgery.

Liposuction is commonly used with breast reduction surgery to ensure that the best shape is obtained for the breast. If liposuction is not done, the breast can look square and boxy.

3

If most of the breast is fatty tissue and excess skin isn't an issue, you can have your breasts reduced in size by **liposuction** alone. For many women, however, this is not an option.

Breast reduction is considered **major surgery** and requires a **general anesthetic**. Surgery takes place in a day surgery clinic or a hospital. Surgery usually takes three to five hours. Depending on the surgeon and clinical setting, you may need to stay overnight (which I highly recommend if possible, as you will need the care of the nursing staff and good pain medication).

There are some cases of smaller reductions only requiring a local anesthetic, but I haven't heard of anyone having a reduction in this manner.

When you see your surgeon, they may recommend a **Breast Lift** instead of a breast reduction. A breast lift can raise sagging or drooping breasts, which as you know is common for heavy breasts, and this will also elevate the nipple and areola. This is a less invasive procedure and usually costs a lot less. But if you want to remove weight and volume, removing a bit of skin and lifting your boobs won't be enough.

The Stats

According to the American Society for Plastic Surgeons (ASAPS), more than 15.6 million cosmetic procedures, including both minimally-invasive and surgical, were performed in the United States in 2014.

Breast reduction surgery is the eighth highest type of cosmetic surgery in the US, with more than 114,470 women undergoing breast reduction surgery in the US in 2014. Due to the rising rates of obesity and often subsequent increases in breast size, this number is set to increase.

According to one study, 80% of women reported that the outcome of their surgery was good or very good.

4

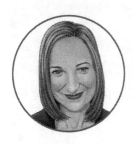

Ayesha: When I saw the first surgeon about a breast reduction, she was very resistant to giving me a breast reduction and only wanted to do a breast lift. When I saw a second surgeon, I realized why she didn't want to give me the reduction. Because of the shape, weight and position of the breast tissue, and the lack of breast tissue in the upper part of my breast, the surgery I required was more complex. I don't think the surgeon I saw first, who I later realized was a general surgeon and not a plastic or cosmetic surgeon, had the skills to do a reduction on me.

"More often than not, the ideal breast is an invented breast. Decolletage, the tushy breast, is an artifact of clothing. Naked breasts don't dance cheek to cheek-- they turn away from each other. Breasts vary in size and shape to an outlandish degree, but they can be whipped into an impressive conformity, and because we are human and we can't leave anything alone, we have whipped away."
Natalie Angier
Writer

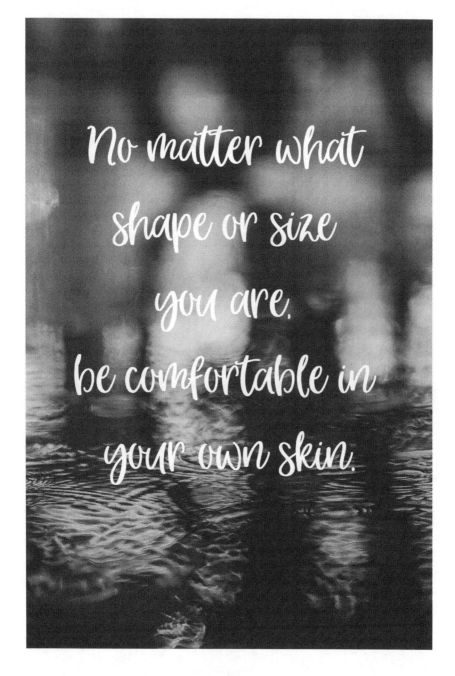

No matter what
shape or size
you are,
be comfortable in
your own skin.

Chapter 2:
Benefits of Breast Reduction Surgery

I have met a lot of women over the last twenty years who have had breast reductions. And the most striking thing is that I have not met anyone who has regretted having their boobs reduced. Even the ones who had issues after their surgery would still prefer to have smaller boobs.

If you're like the women I have spoken with, then you know what it's like to lug around the heavy weight of boobs around your neck and shoulders. You also know how hard it is to find clothes that fit nicely because so many clothes are made for very small breasts.

And then there's the confidence issue. So many of us busty women try not to draw attention to our boobs (while some confident women are great at using these large assets!). We are self-conscious of our buxom chests. I had a lot of unwelcome male attention from "sleaze bags" obsessed with big boobs.

Breast reduction isn't for everyone, but it might suit you if:

- You suffer from **neck**, **back** and **shoulder pain** from having breasts that are too large for your frame

- You have breasts that, due to their weight, **point downwards**

- One of your **breasts is larger than the other**

- You are **self-conscious** about how large your breasts are

- Your breasts limit your **physical activity** (running is not fun when it hurts your chest and you need more than one bra to hold your breasts firmly)

- You suffer skin **irritation** beneath the breast crease

- Your breasts **hang low** and you have **stretched skin**

- You have regular **indentations** on your shoulders from bra straps

- Your **areolas** are **enlarged** due to stretched skin

Benefits of Breast Reduction

There are physical, cosmetic and psychological benefits of breast reduction surgery, including:

- Reduced back and neck pain

- Other physical symptoms, such as headaches, should decrease

- Skin rashes beneath your breast tissue will disappear

- Exercise and physical activity will become more comfortable

- Your breasts will be lifted and firmer

- Your breasts will look more youthful

- Bras will fit more comfortably and attractively

- Your breasts will be more in proportion with the rest of your body

- Stretched areolas and/or large nipples can be reduced

- Swimsuits, sports bras, and clothes will look and feel better

- You will probably have more confidence

Another positive thing is that breast reduction surgery has the highest patient satisfaction rating of all plastic surgery procedures. According to the American Society of Aesthetic Plastic Surgery survey data, women report being happier and healthier emotionally, physically and sexually after breast reduction surgery.

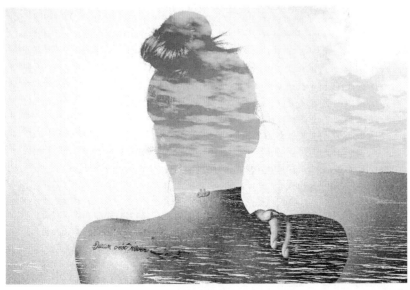

Jane's Story

My breasts had been depressing me for years. I come from a family of women who all have extremely large breasts. I had back problems, constant headaches, and neck pain. I couldn't stand up for long periods because of the pain, so I spent my life looking for a place to sit down.

I was embarrassed by how my breasts looked naked. They were saggy due to the weight of the breast and the nipples pointed down. I had been single for years, and I was too shy to date because of my breasts. The thought of a man seeing me naked horrified me.

I would have loved to have had surgery when I was younger, but I didn't have the money, and my insurance wouldn't cover it. When I finally had the money to pay for a private surgeon, I ended up going with the first surgeon I met with. I knew straight away that he was the right one for me. He specialized in breast reduction and was skilled at working with women with extremely large breasts like me.

My surgery went as planned. I didn't have any complications. The recovery was harder than I expected. I was very tired and needed more rest than I anticipated. My mother helped care for me, so at least I had some support.

I had over three and a half pounds removed from each breast. I went from an H cup to a DD. I can't tell you how much of a difference it has made to my life. I am more active, I sleep better, and I am starting to date for the first time in years.

CHAPTER 3

Risks of Breast Reduction Surgery

Modern surgery is generally safe, though it always carries a risk; complications can and do occur. Most of the women I have spoken with did not experience any complications, though I know of one poor woman who had to have repeated corrective surgery when her nipple and areola died, which sounded very traumatic.

While I knew the risks going into my surgery, for me the benefits of the surgery outweighed the risks. For some women, the risk is too high. And if you're a smoker or have other health complications, then the risks may not be worth the benefits.

Only you can make that decision, in consultation with your surgeon, but you do need to know the potential worst-case scenarios.

General Surgery Risks

Many of the risks involved in breast reduction surgery are the same as those for any major surgery and include:

- Risks of having general anesthesia, such as **allergic reaction** and potentially fatal cardiovascular complications such as a **heart attack**

- Surgical risks such as **bleeding** or **infection**

- **Breathing difficulties** due to the general anesthetic or the tube that is put down your through (endotracheal tube) which can cause swelling, discomfort and loud breathing

- A **blood clot** in the veins of your legs (deep vein thrombosis) which can move to the lungs (pulmonary embolus) or the brain, and may be life threatening

- **Fluid accumulation** at the site of the surgery

- **Allergic reaction** to the suture materials, adhesive tape or other medical materials

- **Skin** discoloration, permanent pigmentation changes, swelling and bruising

- **Damage** to blood vessels, nerves, muscles, and lungs (this can be temporary or permanent)

- Fatty tissue deep in the skin could die (this is called **fat necrosis**)

Breast Reduction Surgery Risks

The additional risks and complications specifically for breast reduction include:

- Changes in breast and nipple **sensation** (this is one of the things that women fear the most)

- Temporary or permanent areas of **numbness**

- **Asymmetry** (unevenness) of the breasts

- Potential partial or total **loss of nipple and areola** (this one is the scariest to me – the risk of the nipple and areola dying)

- **Severe scarring** (some women do have extreme scarring in the form of Keloid Scarring – this means that the scars are raised, often itchy, and do not heal like normal

scars)

- Some women experience **fat necrosis**, where the fat clumps together

- **Wound healing problems** – sometimes a wound will tear open and fail to heal easily (this happened to me and was quite scary)

- Possible need for **revision** surgery or procedures to fix issues (such as "dog ears" – I have these and did not get them fixed)

If any of these complications happen, then you might have to undergo further surgery to treat the problem. Some issues, though, like reduced breast sensation or numbness, may not be treatable at all.

While there are no guarantees with any surgery, these risks can be minimized by choosing a properly trained and qualified surgeon as well as following their advice before and after surgery.

See *Chapter 19: Post-Op Breasts* for more information on what you may experience after surgery.

Other Considerations

Here are some things to consider that may impact your decision to have a breast reduction:

- If you are **young** and your breasts are still developing, it is best to wait until your breasts are fully developed (it's often recommended to wait until your early to mid-20s).

- If you still plan to have **children** and **breastfeed**, surgeons generally recommend waiting until after this phase of life to have your reduction.

- If you have a significant amount of **weight** to lose, it is better to get to your ideal weight before surgery, as changes in weight will impact your breast size.

- If you **smoke**, you are at increased risk of complications, so if you're planning to quit anyway, use your breast reduction as a motivator to quit smoking.

- If you have breast or nipple **piercings**, these can cause infection.

Have Realistic Expectations

By reading this book, you are educating yourself about the breast reduction process. The whole aim of this book is to prepare you so that you know what to expect at the various stages of your breast reduction. If you know what to expect, you are more empowered to make the right decisions for you. And you will have less stress and disappointment.

Your Breasts Won't Look Like Breast Augmentation

I'm sure you know what augmented, or surgically enlarged, breasts look like. They are perky things that sit high on the chest.

The truth is your breasts probably won't look like this. However, your breasts will probably have quite a natural look and feel to them. If you are after super pert breasts, this can sometimes be achieved with reduction surgery. However, you want to be realistic in your expectations.

You Need to Be Patient

Your breasts will take a long time to heal and settle into their new shape. Some women find their breasts don't normalize until 12 months after surgery.

There Will Be Scars

Breast reduction surgery has evolved since it was first developed in the 1950's. The procedure today is more sophisticated, resulting in less scarring. However, there is no way to avoid scars unless you are having a liposuction-only breast reduction.

Educate Yourself

Read this whole book before you make a definite decision about having breast reduction surgery.

Talina's Story

I'm happy with the outcome of my surgery, smaller breasts, but the experience itself was quite traumatic. I don't take a lot of medication, so when I was signing the release forms before my surgery, I struggled to tick the box that said I would agree to all and any medications being administered for any reasons. What I really wanted was to give my consent to any medication. I felt like I couldn't advocate on my behalf and it was out of my control, and I would have no recourse because I signed the form.

Perhaps it was my intuition warning me because I had an overdose while in surgery. The anesthesiologist gave me too much anesthesia and I started to crash. They did tests to find out what was going on and they charged me for them even though they had created the problem in the first place.

I was very ill after surgery because of the overdose; however, the emotional impact was far more scarring. I didn't realize it until a few months later, but I had experienced a form of post-traumatic stress. Even now, six months later, I feel sick when I think about the surgery, my heart beats faster and I feel hot and sweaty.

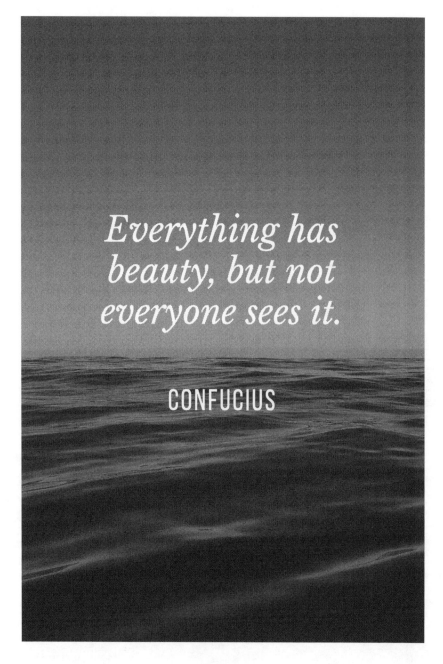

Everything has beauty, but not everyone sees it.

CONFUCIUS

CHAPTER 4

Anatomy of Breasts

You and I have breasts, but that doesn't mean we really understand how they work! I don't remember learning much about breasts in high school biology (it would have been mortifying in a co-ed school).

It is important to understand the anatomy of the breast so that you can understand what's involved in breast reduction surgery. Let's find out a little more about these amazing mammary glands.

Mammary Glands

Breasts, also known as mammary glands, are only found in mammals – thus why they are called mammary glands. They are an exocrine gland that produces milk to feed offspring. In humans, the mammary glands take the form of breasts. In cows, deer, and goats, they take the form of udders. And in dogs and cats, mammary glands are known as dugs. Of course, we are only interested in human breasts here.

Mammal embryos start out along a continuum of development pathway that has the potential to produce male or female anatomy. As the embryo grows, sex-specific hormones are produced and determine whether the embryo becomes a male or a female. A female embryo will develop female sex organs, including breast glands.

Anatomy of Your Breast

The breast is the tissue overlying the chest (pectoral) muscles. A woman's breast is made up of glandular tissue (that produces milk when lactating) and fatty tissue. It is the amount of fatty tissue that determines the size of the breast. Younger women often have denser, less fatty, breast tissue than older women who have gone through menopause.

Glandular tissue has 15 to 20 sections called **lobes** that branch out from the nipple. Each lobe is made up of smaller structures, called **lobules** that produce milk when a woman is lactating. Each lobule holds tiny, hollow sacs called **alveoli**. When breastfeeding, milk travels through a network of tiny tubes called **ducts** from the alveoli. These ducts connect and join together into larger ducts. The larger ducts then connect to the **nipple** and allow milk to exit.

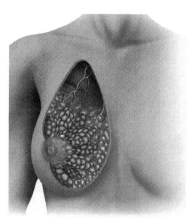

Spaces around the lobules and ducts are filled with fat, ligaments and connective tissue. **Ligaments** and **connective tissue** provide support to the breast and give it shape.

Sensation in the breast occurs via **nerves**. Oxygen and nutrients travel to breast tissue through the blood in your arteries and capillaries (thin, fragile blood vessels).

The breast structure also includes the lymphatic system, which is a network of lymph nodes and lymph ducts that help fight infection. Lymph nodes are found under the armpit, above the collarbone, behind the breastbone and in other parts of the body. They trap harmful substances that may be in the lymphatic system and safely drain them from the body.

The breast has no muscle, except for some tiny muscles in

the nipple. There is muscle between the breast and your rib cage.

The dark area around the nipple, as you probably know, is the **areola**. The purpose of the areola is two-fold: it helps support the nipple, and it contains Montgomery's glands which keep the nipple moisturized during breastfeeding.

Nearly all women have the same milk-producing structures within their breasts. As you know, women's breast tissue is sensitive to cyclic changes in hormone levels, and that is why women often experience sore and tender breasts just before and during menstruation.

Your breasts change over the course of your life. They may get bigger during pregnancy. They will often get smaller when you lose weight and increase in size when you gain weight.

Please see *Chapter 25: Weight Changes & Your Breast Size Post-Surgery* for more information on how changes in your weight will affect your breasts.

Please see *Chapter 12: Breastfeeding After Breast Reduction* for more information on how breast reduction impacts breastfeeding.

Female Breast Anatomy

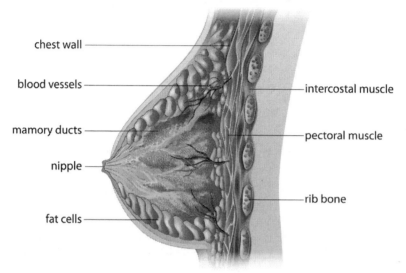

chest wall
blood vessels
mamory ducts
nipple
fat cells
intercostal muscle
pectoral muscle
rib bone

Drew Barrymore's Breast Reduction

I've always been a fan of actress Drew Barrymore. In 1992, at the age of 17, Drew had a breast reduction. She's been quoted as saying: "There's something very awkward about women and their breasts because men look at them so much. When they're huge, you become very self-conscious. Your back hurts. You find that whatever you wear, you look heavy in. It's uncomfortable."

Tonya's Story

I had breast reduction surgery just over a year ago. OMG! I wish I had done it sooner. I developed breasts at a young age. My mom said I had small breast mounds as young as seven. Even before I hit my teens, I was wearing a bra. By the time I was in high school, I was a C cup. As I matured, my breasts continued to grow. They eventually stopped at an FF cup.

My friends and I would often go shopping after school. They were able to buy bras off the shelf at Target and Kmart. I had to have mine ordered through the lingerie shop. My bras were ugly. They looked like something my grandmother would wear. They were normally very plain, as big as a sack, and beige. I longed for pretty bras!

Thankfully, due to my large cup size and my small frame, I was able to get my insurance to cover the cost of the surgery. I was only 19 when I had surgery. Ideally, I should have waited until I was a few years older, but I just couldn't.

I was scared on the day of surgery. I've never broken a bone, stayed in hospital or even had stitches. Luckily my mom was with me. My surgeon was lovely as well. She made me feel safe and explained everything to me.

Recovery was tough. I didn't feel good. I looked even worse. But I had no regrets. Not one. One of the first things I did after my breast reduction was throw out all my bras and undies. I bought all matching bra and knickers.

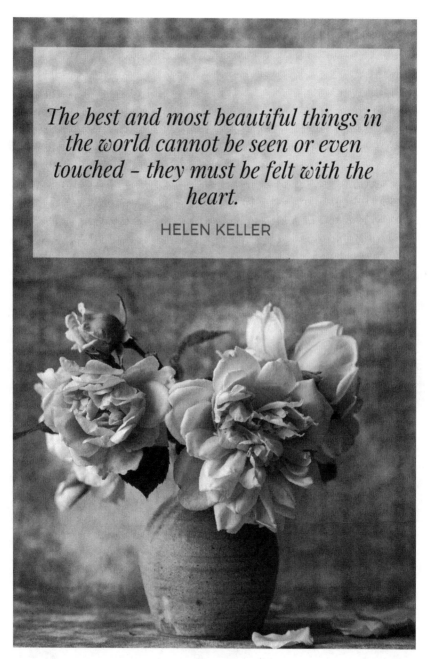

The best and most beautiful things in the world cannot be seen or even touched – they must be felt with the heart.

HELEN KELLER

CHAPTER 5

Breast Reduction Techniques - Overview

There are several common breast reduction techniques. While you may have a preference for the type of breast reduction you want, the technique your surgeon suggests will depend on a number of factors.

Factors that influence the type of surgery suitable for you, and will give you the best outcome include:

- Your breast size

- The amount of tissue to be removed

- The shape of your breast

- Whether you want to breastfeed in the future

- The surgeon's preference and expertise

Modern breast reduction surgery usually uses one of these three techniques:

1. **Pedicle Method (with Many Different Variations)**
   The pedicle method maintains blood and nerve flow to the nipple and areola during surgery. This helps retain nipple sensation and function.

   There are two main times of pedicle surgery:
   Vertical/Lollipop Method
   Extends around the top of the areola with a V-shaped

incision down the midline of the breast.

Anchor/Inverted T Method
Extends around the top of the areola and down across the lower portion of the breast. The nipple and areola remain attached to blood and nerve supply and are moved up once the underlying breast tissue is removed.

2. Free Nipple Graft
The nipple and areola are removed during surgery and then replaced after the breast tissue has been removed.

3. Liposuction-Only Breast Reduction
Liposuction is used to reduce fatty tissue from the breast.

Most women have a bilateral breast reduction where both breasts are reduced. Women who have one breast noticeably larger than the other, may opt to have a unilateral reduction where only one breast is reduced.

Incisions for breast reduction surgery will result in a scar around the areola and a vertical line extending down to the bottom of the breast. This may or may not be accompanied by a scar along the bottom of the breast line.

Techniques that do not involve the vertical scar (which many women worry about) will generally not bring the best result, especially for those with quite large breasts.

One question you need to ask yourself, then, what is more important to you? The shape of your breast? Or a scar that will fade over time?

When thinking about which technique is best for you, your surgeon should factor in what is most important to you, whether it is fullness up top, removing bulk, or the size you're ultimately aiming for.

As I will say throughout this book, you should consult with at least three surgeons to compare their recommendations. If you're not happy with the method a surgeon is suggesting, get another opinion, especially if they are recommending a free nipple graft. Take the time, and put in the effort, to find the best surgeon and surgical procedure for you.

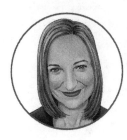

Ayesha: My breast reduction was more complicated than some, due to the amount of excess skin I had on my breasts post-breastfeeding. The first surgeon I saw didn't want to do a breast reduction at all and said I only needed a lift. I wonder now if this was because her skill level was not up to the task. She was a general surgeon, not a cosmetic surgeon.

Clarissa's Story

I've always been self-conscious about my breasts. I developed large breasts in high school. I think I was in year eight and I was wearing a DD bra. I stopped playing sport because I was so uncomfortable physically. I didn't like the attention I got from boys at school, who would tease me about my breasts (you can imagine what year eight and nine boys are like).

So, I stopped wearing tight clothes. My uniform became baggy tops, loose jackets, and scarves. Wearing a scarf made me feel like I was hiding my breasts from the world and I developed a good collection of scarves.

Most of my friends, even ones I have had for years, had no idea that I had big breasts because I always hid them. I knew that dressing like this made me look heavier than I was, but disguising my breasts was more important to me than looking slim.

I had a breast reduction about a year ago. The only people that knew were my husband, my children, and my parents. My breasts have healed really well and I love how small they are (I'm a B to C cup depending on the bra). My body confidence is slowly improving. I have even started wearing dresses. I've not shown my cleavage yet, but I am working towards it. I've spent 20 years hiding my body and now I am learning to enjoy it.

CHAPTER 6

Breast Reduction Techniques
- Pedicle Method

The Pedicle Method is the most commonly performed breast reduction procedure. A breast pedicle is the areola and nipple area (known as the areola complex) attached to tissues that are still connected to blood supply, nerves, and milk ducts.

The pedicle method reduces breast appearance, volume, and contour, while maintaining breast function and nipple sensation. This method is very safe because it does not sever blood flow, milk duct functioning or nerves.

In the pedicle method, the nipple will be re-positioned to a more aesthetically pleasing place on the body. This involves cutting around the areola complex, often in its entirety. The areola complex remains connected to tissue, blood supply and ducts. If performed correctly, pedicle techniques should allow you to breastfeed following your surgery, but there are no guarantees.

In breast reduction, a pedicle can be either from above the areola (superior pedicle), to one side of the areola (medial pedicle from close to the center or lateral pedicle from the outside of the breast), below the areola (inferior pedicle), or directly underneath the areola complex (central pedicle). These are explained in more detail later.

There are two main types of pedicle methods used in breast reduction surgery, the Vertical or Lollipop Method and the Inverted-T or Anchor Breast Reduction.

Vertical or Lollipop Breast Reduction

The vertical short scar or lollipop breast reduction is most commonly used on women who require a moderate reduction and only have mild sagging. This method is relatively new and is gaining in popularity due to the decrease in scarring compared with the Anchor Method (see below).

For women with breasts with a DD or less, this can be a good option. You need to have good skin elasticity for this method, with not a lot of breast tissue needing to be removed.

The Vertical Method is also known as Vertical Mammoplasty, VOQ, Vertical, and Regnought, LeJour Method.

The surgery involves two incision sites, one around the edge of the areola and a second running vertically from the bottom of the areola to the crease beneath the breast (the inframammary fold).

This incision pattern allows the surgeon to remove excess fat, skin and breast tissue, reshape the breast internally, and lift the breast into a more youthful position. Some surgeons may do a modified version of this method where they add very short horizontal incision on either side of the vertical incision to help shape the breasts.

This method does leave scarring, but the scars are not visible when wearing a bra as the scars are below the nipple.

The name lollipop is often used for this surgery because the scars are in the shape of a lollipop – a circle on a stick!

[Insert Image of Vertical Reduction]

Anchor or Inverted-T Breast Reduction

The Anchor, or Inverted-T, is also known by a lot of other names, including Bilateral Reduction Mammoplasty, T-Scar,

T-Incision, McKissock, and the Weiss Method.

The anchor reduction involves three incisions; one a round circular shape around the edge of the areola, one vertically from the areola down the front of the breast to the breast crease, and one made along the crease underneath the breast (this third incision is the major difference between this and the vertical/lollipop method).

The anchor technique allows for the maximum degree of tissue removal and reshaping, so surgeons will typically use this approach if a patient needs a more significant breast size reduction, and/or has considerable sagging or asymmetry to correct.

The scars resulting from an inverted-T or anchor breast reduction are similar to those from a vertical reduction, but with one additional, thin scar running along the crease beneath the breast. Like the vertical technique, the scars are contained below the nipple, so can be easily concealed beneath bras, swimsuits, and clothing.

[Insert Image of Anchor Reduction]

Stevens Laser Bra

I wanted to mention the Stevens Laser Bra. It is a very new and innovative approach to breast surgery. It was created by Dr. W. Grand Stevens, a plastic surgeon in the US. The Stevens Laser Bra creates an internal bra using your own tissue. It apparently makes breasts look and feel younger longer.

The incision patterns are the same as with most of the anchor style pedicle methods, along with preservation of the pedicle, so that nipple function and sensation are retained.

Dr. Stevens says, *"The whole point of The Stevens Laser Bra is to create a beautiful, longer-lasting and more permanent lift of the breasts to enhance breast lift and breast reduction surgeries."*

It seems to be solely practiced in Beverly Hills at Dr. Stevens' clinic. For more information, see: www.laserbra.com.

Different Pedicle Techniques to Maintain Blood & Nerve Supply

Pedicle techniques are often defined as inferior, superior, central, lateral or bi-pedicle. These are ascribed according to the way the blood and nerves are maintained from different areas of the breast:

- Inferior Pedicle

- Superior Pedicle

- Central/Medial Pedicle

- Lateral Pedicle

- Bi-Pedicle

Clarify with your surgeon what they mean when they describe surgery as pedicle as well as determine exactly which type of pedicle technique they would be using.

Inferior Pedicle – Bottom of the Breast

This is the most commonly used pedicle method and it maintains the blood and nerve supply from the bottom of the breast. The inferior pedicle has been popular since the mid-1970s. Many surgeons prefer this pedicle because of the relative ease of the surgery. The main complication of the inferior technique is bottoming out. (See *Chapter 19: Post-Op Breasts* for more information on bottoming out.)

Superior Pedicle – Top of the Breast

The superior pedicle method maintains the blood and nerve

supply from the top of the breast. Like the inferior pedicle, the superior pedicle has been commonly used since the 1970s. The superior pedicle gives upper breast fullness and good breast projection and is usually used for women who do not have very large breasts (less than 1 kilo or 5 pounds of breast tissue to be removed). This technique has higher rates of sensation loss than the inferior pedicle technique.

Central– Centre of Breast

The central pedicle maintains the blood and nerve supply from the center of the breast. This technique allows women to retain nipple sensation and function. It is used for very large breasts and is a good alternative to the free nipple graft (see *Chapter 7: Free Nipple Graft* for more information on why you want to avoid a nipple graft).

Lateral Pedicle – Outer Side of Breast

The lateral pedicle maintains the blood and nerve supply from the side of the breast. This type of pedicle is less commonly used and may be considered when most of the tissue to be removed lies in the underside and middle of the breast. Sometimes, this kind of pedicle is also used for a breast lift.

Bi-Pedicle – Top & Bottom of Breast

The bi-pedicle maintains the blood and nerve supply from both the superior/top and inferior/bottom locations. A pedicle is made that points either down and outward, or down and inward. This is a slight variation on the superior pedicle technique.

Maria's Story

It's sad for me to admit, but there was never a time I liked
my breasts. In fact, I hated them. Before I had breasts, I
was mad at them because they took so long to catch up to
my friends. Then I was mad at them because they didn't stop
growing at a reasonable size. I went from a C cup to a D cup,
then to an E cup.

I know many women with small boobs who'd love bigger
ones. I know my small breasted friends wanted breasts like
mine. It was weird because they wanted what I had and I
would have happily have had their smaller boobs. Some of
my friends even had breast enlargements.

The sheer weight of my breasts created poor posture and I
was ashamed of my breasts because they were so large. I
never stood up straight. I would hunch over, caving my chest
inwards, ruining my posture. And the bra straps would dig
into my shoulders leaving indents and red marks.

My breasts were not only enormous; they were also covered
in stretch marks. I felt like I looked fatter than I was because
of my breasts. And I had to buy larger sized clothes that fitted my breasts but not the rest of me.

One day I was lamenting the size of my breasts to a new
friend. She told me how she'd had a breast reduction a few
months before I met her. My friend was very happy with her
breasts. She told me all about her surgery and even showed
me her scars.

I spoke to my mom about breast reduction surgery and she fully supported me. She came to all my appointments with me. I found a good surgeon in my area. I wasn't able to get my surgery covered by insurance, so my Mum and Dad paid for it. It was the best present ever.

I love shopping now. I used to hate it. But best of all, I feel more confident. I'm not as shy as I used to be. And I hardly ever get a sore neck or headaches anymore.

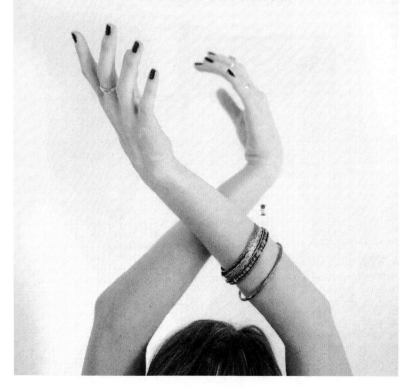

The best preparation for tomorrow is doing your best today.

H. JACKSON BROWN. JR.

CHAPTER 7

Breast Reduction Techniques
- Free Nipple Graft (FNG)

A Free Nipple Graft (FNG) sounds a bit scary, doesn't it? An FNG involves removing the nipple completely and grafting it in its new location as a skin graft. Sensation and function are lost when you have an FNG. Your nipple will not become erect when stimulated and it will feel numb.

The pedicle method is the ideal way to have a breast reduction because the whole pedicle area (the nipple and areola) remains intact, maintaining blood and nerve supply. This preserves function and sensation.

However, there are some instances where FNG may be required if the breasts are extremely large and pendulous. An FNG may be required when the notch-to-nipple measurement is great than 40 centimeters (15 inches) and/or the fold to nipple measurement is great than 20 centimeters (7.5 inches).

Many FNGs are performed unnecessarily by surgeons who do not have very good breast reduction skills. Highly skilled surgeons can often avoid FNGs even with extremely large breasts.

If your surgeon recommends an FNG, you want to make sure they have a good reason for doing so. And you can always get a second or third opinion (which I highly recommend). You don't want to lose nipple sensation and function if you don't have to.

Warning: If you have an FNG done and require more breast surgery in the future, be certain to tell the surgeon. It is easy to mistake an FNG for a pedicle method reduction, especially if you had a highly skilled surgeon. If your new surgeon doesn't know you've had an FNG, they might destroy the blood supply to the area where you had the graft, and this could destroy your nipples and areola. You do not want to risk causing the death of your nipples.

FNG Process

Here is the FNG process:

1. The nipple and areola are removed swiftly and placed on a moist saline sponge

2. The surgeon removes most of the breast tissue

3. A pocket is made of the skin, and the remaining breast tissue is put in the pocket

4. The skin is trimmed to size, shaped around the breast, and then stitched together

5. Once the breast is reformed, the nipple and areola are grafted into place

Scar Pattern

There is no pedicle in an FNG because there is no blood supply from the breast itself. As with other skin grafts, the blood supply comes from the deep dermis. The scar pattern of an FNG reduction will most likely look like an anchor pattern. However, do clarify this with your surgeon.

Risks of an FNG

The risks of a Free Nipple Graft include:

- The surgeon removes too much breast tissue and the breast cannot be shaped properly

- The nipple and areola may look unnatural

- The nipple and areola may not survive the grafting process

- The color of the nipple and areola may fade due to the grafting process (there is a higher risk of this happening for darker skin)

- The nipple will most likely lose all sensation

- The nipple will no longer become erect when stimulated

- Breastfeeding is impossible due to the milk ducts being severed, removed, or rearranged

- Should be avoided in young women, especially those who would like to breastfeed

- If nipple sensation and function are important, an FNG will not be suitable for you

Benefits of an FNG

Given the risks of a Free Nipple Graft, you may be wondering why a surgeon would recommend one at all. Here are some of the reasons:

- It is a relatively quick surgery, so time under anesthesia is reduced

- There is minimal blood loss

- Better shaping for extremely large breasts – if large amounts of tissue need to be removed, it can be difficult to protect the pedicle and shape the breast properly

- May allow for a smaller breast size to be reached than would be possible with other methods

37

There are a lot of unnecessary FNGs done today. While some are necessary due to the size of a woman's breasts, an unskilled plastic surgeon may do these routinely and think this is acceptable. It is not. You would want to avoid an unnecessary FNG with an unskilled plastic surgeon.

Melissa's Story

I come from a family of large-breasted women. My grandmother, my mother, my aunts, and my sisters all have enormous breasts. We are tall, big-boned people. There are no petite women in my family. I was used to big breasts and they were something to be celebrated in my family. At family gatherings, someone would always make a joke about breasts. We were able to laugh at our bosoms.

Even despite this positive appreciation of large breasts, I really wanted to get a breast reduction. No one in my family had ever had one. I talked to my mom and sisters about it. At first, they were surprised, but once we talked about it, they were really supportive.

I went from an H cup down to a D cup. It was a huge change for me. At first, my breasts felt so small compared to what they used to be. I didn't feel like myself at first, but I soon got used to them. Now I love them. They have a great shape, very natural, and they are so light. I no longer feel like I am wearing two kilos of rice around my neck.

Since I had my surgery, one of my sisters also had a reduction. My mum is thinking about getting one too. She's a bit older and I think she thinks it isn't worth it at her age. I told her to go for it because she will feel so much more comfortable.

CHAPTER 8

Breast Reduction Techniques - Liposuction-Only

Some women will be able to have a liposuction-only breast reduction. This type of breast reduction creates the least amount of scarring. Many people think there is no scaring, but small incisions are made on the breasts where lipcannula are inserted. These incisions will obviously scar like any wound. However, the scarring is minimal.

The Liposuction-Only Breast Reduction Process

Here is the normal process for a liposuction breast reduction:

1. Normally done as an outpatient procedure at a hospital or day surgery clinic

2. You will be hooked up to an IV which will deliver sedation

3. Two incisions are made in each breast

4. Fluid is injected into each breast to separate the tissue from the fat

5. Liposuction is performed on each breast

Advantages of Liposuction-Only Breast Reduction

There are a number of advantages and benefits to liposuction-only breast reduction, including:

- Minimal scars

- Doesn't require general anesthetic

- Minimal blood loss

- Does not change the nipple and areola

- Done as a day procedure

- Quicker and less invasive than breast reduction surgery

- May be cheaper than surgical breast reduction

- Can be less painful and have a shorter recovery time

- The results are normally lasting

Disadvantages of Liposuction-Only Breast Reduction

There are a number of disadvantages and risks to liposuction-only breast reduction, including:

- Only effective for women who want a small reduction

- Does not address sagging, asymmetrical breasts, or stretched skin

- There is no lifting of the breast

- Can create a "deflated balloon" effect

- Breast tissue may become more dense

- There is no change to the areola (if you have a large areola and would like it made smaller, you can only get that with surgical reduction)

- Some women report extreme pain with liposuction and may take as long to recover as women who have surgical breast reduction

- Many women who have lipo-only are dissatisfied with the results and end up having a breast reduction and lift later

Jacinta's Story

I was quite skinny growing up, and I didn't have any boobs to speak of for most of the way through high school. I also got my period later than my friends. When I was about 17, I started to put on weight. Almost overnight, I went from a skinny flat chested girl to a plump one with size D breasts.

At first, I didn't mind having bigger boobs; I was excited to have cleavage! But as I struggled with my weight and con-tinued to get heavier, so did my boobs. Before long, I had constant headaches and my neck was always stiff. I wore a bodysuit for years to help spread the weight out and reduce the pain.

I had thought about breast reduction for quite a few years before I had one. I was nervous about having surgery. And I also wanted to breastfeed. After I had finished breastfeeding my third child, I decided that it was time for me to finally get a breast reduction.

I was still overweight, but I couldn't wait until I lost weight (if I ever did). I have thyroid problems, and I am on medication, but it isn't helping me lose weight. My breasts were very sag-ging after breastfeeding for over four years.

I shopped around for a surgeon. I didn't feel comfortable with the first two I met. They seemed arrogant and didn't really listen to me. The third surgeon I tried was great. She answered all my questions. Her office helped me fill out the paperwork for my insurer.

Before my surgery, I was an H cup. I wanted to go down to a C or a D cup if I could. My surgeon was able to remove more than 2 kilos of breast tissue. I went down to a D cup, and I couldn't have been happier. I have a scar around my nipple, one down the front of my breast, and one underneath. I'm not worried about the scars at my age. I'm just happy to have smaller breasts. I can even wear clothes at home without a bra. That's freedom! And as an added bonus, my breasts are more pert than ever.

CHAPTER 9

Scarring

Scarring is one of the biggest concerns of women thinking of having a reduction. As this is major invasive surgery, scarring is inevitable. A good surgeon will try to minimize the scarring and make the scars along the natural folds of your breasts.

If you think of skin as a seamless organ, it is a like a precious fine cloth protecting you. If that cloth was made of silk, just one small tear can make a difference to how it looks. Imagine then if you stitched up this tear in this beautiful silk cloth. Depending on the cloth and the way it has been stitched, chances are you would still be able to identify where the tear was.

This is the same for skin. The fact is that a scar will never go away completely. When you have breast reduction surgery, there will be scarring. However, there are ways to reduce scarring.

Scars and healing after your breast reduction surgery depend on a number of factors, including:

- The type of surgery

- How you normally heal from trauma to the skin

- Your overall health

- As well as how you care for your breasts after surgery

Scar Locations

The location of the scars will depend on the type of breast reduction technique used. The scars are generally not visible when you wear a normal bra. Like any scar, they will fade over time. If you are prone to scarring, as some women are, please let your surgeon know.

Laser Scar Treatment

About six weeks after your surgery, your surgeon may have you assessed for laser treatment for your scarring. This can speed up the recovery process by causing new skin to grow more quickly. Laser may not be suitable for all scarring. Some surgeons include a complimentary laser treatment in their overall breast reduction plan.

Keloid Scars

I didn't really know much about this until someone I know developed severe keloid scarring following her breast reduc-tion. Keloid scarring meant that she developed thick scar tissue along the surgical lines. Whereas my scars continue to fade, this woman's scars are raised, often itchy, and are not decreasing in size. This woman also had laser treatment for her scarring, which may have made it worse (this is not a proven fact, but given her risk factor for keloid scarring, it does make me wonder).

I must admit that when I saw the severity of this scarring, I was shocked, and I had tears in my eyes. I was upset for her, especially as she had done everything she could possibly do to reduce the scar tissue.

Think about how you scar. Do your scars fade quite easily or do they pucker up and leave raised scar tissue? How you have scarred in the past will be a fair indicator of how your scars will heal post-surgery.

If you're not sure about whether you've had Keloid Scaring,

44

look it up on the internet to see various images. You may also want to mention to your surgeon if you've had problems with scarring or wound healing in the past. Please note, that keloid scarring is more common on darker skin.

See *Chapter 20: Minimizing Scar Tissue* for more information on how to minimize scar tissues.

Rose's Story

For years, I harbored a secret wish to have a breast reduction. One day, I decided to talk to my boyfriend, Rob, about it. We'd been dating for about 18 months and had recently moved in together. I'd just got a promotion at work and I had really good health coverage. I broached the idea of breast reduction with Rob one night as we ate dinner.

He nearly choked on his pasta. He said, "Babe, I love your boobs. Why would you want to make them smaller? Do you know how many women would love to have breasts like yours?"

I was shocked. I thought he would be more supportive. I shelved the idea and didn't bring it up again for a long time. Then Rob asked me to marry him. I was over the moon.

I went wedding dress shopping with my best friend, Sophie. After going to a couple of different shops, I started to feel really down. I couldn't find a single dress that fitted and looked any good. Most were strapless, which doesn't work when you're an FF cup.

Over coffee after the dress shopping debacle, I told Sophie that I really wanted a breast reduction and how Rob didn't want me to have one. Sophie is a straight talker, that's one of the reasons I love her, and she said to me, "Rose, it's your body. You're the one who has to carry these boobs around. I'm sure Rob will come on board if you get a reduction."

Sophie was right. It was my body and I didn't need anyone's approval or permission to do what I wanted – which was to have a breast reduction.

I spoke with Rob about it. I told him how hard it was all the time – not being able to find clothes that fit, having men look at my breasts instead of my face, being uncomfortable and in pain, and not finding a beautiful wedding dress.

Rob was a lot more supportive after I shared all this with him. He even apologized for not being supportive last time. Rob came to all my appointments with me and took good care of me after my surgery. He took time off work and we watched a lot of Netflix shows together.

My breast reduction surgery created a deeper bond between Rob and me, and I'm happier than ever that this is the man I get to spend my life with. I had my surgery six months ago and I'm getting married next month. I have the most gorgeous wedding dress. It's strapless and shows off my new breasts beautifully.

CHAPTER 10

Costs & Insurance

Alas, the decision to have a breast reduction may come down to money. Breast reduction surgery isn't cheap. Many women have to put off surgery for a long time due to the costs of surgery being outside their reach. The costs of surgery will vary depending on a number of factors. If you have insurance, you still may have a battle on your hands to get your breast reduction surgery covered.

Breast Reduction Costs

Costs can vary a lot depending on the surgeon, whether you have health insurance that covers breast reduction, and whether you are in a public or private hospital.

The cost of the surgeon can be influenced by the experience and qualifications of the surgeon, the type of breast reduction procedure required, and even the geographic location of the surgeon's office.

Generally, the cost of a breast reduction would include:

- Surgeon's fee (for appointments and surgery)

- Hospital or surgical facility costs

- Anesthesia fees

- Prescriptions for medication

- Post-surgery garments

* Medical tests

Health Insurance

Disclaimer: I'm no expert in health insurance. Speak to your doctor or surgeon and your insurance company. The information provided here is based on research I have undertaken.

Breast reduction surgery used to be considered a reconstructive procedure and was often covered by private health insurance. In Australia, health insurance providers are making it more and more difficult to get this procedure covered. Similarly, in the US, it can be quite challenging to get your breast reduction surgery covered by insurance.

Each individual insurance provider has specific criteria that must be met in order to consider coverage for breast reduction surgery. Check with your insurance company to see if your policy covers breast reduction. Often you can find these criteria on your insurance company's website or by contacting them. Your surgeon's office should also be able to help you determine if your insurance will cover you and guide you in getting the appropriate paperwork in order. You may, however, need to jump through a few hoops to get covered!

Read Your Policy

Have a good read of your insurance policy. If your insurer lists reduction mammoplasty as policy exclusion, you may not even get coverage for a consultation to discuss whether surgery is appropriate for your symptoms.

Schnur Sliding Scale Chart

Whether insurance will cover breast reduction is often dependent on the size of your breast and the amount of breast tissue to be removed. Many insurance companies use the Schnur Sliding Scale chart to evaluate whether they will cover breast reduction surgery. The scale or formula was

48

developed by Dr. Paul Schnur, a Mayo Clinic-affiliated plastic surgeon, in 1991 who was studying women who'd had breast reduction for medical reasons.

The formula takes into account the patient's body surface area (BSA) and the average weight of breast tissue to be removed. Each insurance provider has a certain number of grams required for removal before they will approve surgery. Often, if the BSA and weight of breast tissue fall below the 22nd percentile, the surgery is deemed as cosmetic and not medically required.

As you can imagine, insurance companies will try hard not to pay for breast reduction surgery, and it is harder than ever to get covered. Even though small breast reductions can make a big difference to a woman's life, insurance companies often only cover big breast reductions, such as going from an F cup to a C cup.

Some policies also consider your height and your weight. If you are petite with a large bust, this may work in your favor. If you are overweight, it may be harder to get coverage.

A 2013 report by Koltz, Fy and Langstein in the Plastic and Reconstructive Journal showed that 86% of insurance providers surveyed still used the 1991 Schnur Sliding Scale to determine whether they would cover breast reduction surgery.

The Schnur chart is an outdated way of calculating whether a woman should be covered for breast reduction surgery. Medical literature has shown that the chart is often used to discriminate against overweight women and deny them coverage because of where they fall on the scale – regardless of their symptoms. These companies fail to consider the last two decades of medical literature that proves the effectiveness of breast reduction surgery in alleviating symptoms of large breasts regardless of a woman's weight.

The Schnur Sliding Scale Chart

Body Surface Area (meters squared)	Minimum weight of tissue to be removed per breast (grams)
1.35	199
1.40	218
1.45	238
1.50	260
1.55	284
1.60	310
1.65	338
1.70	370
1.75	404
1.80	441
1.85	482
1.90	527
1.95	575
2.00	628
2.05	687
2.10	750
2.15	819
2.20	895
2.25	978
2.30 or greater	>= 1000

Interestingly, Dr. Schnur, who developed the Schnur chart, even challenged insurance carriers about the use of the scale to determine coverage, suggesting the scale may not be as useful these days in calculating coverage. He published an article in 1999, in the Annals of Plastic Surgery, to set the record straight. He had found in the years since he published the scale; many insurers were misusing the scale to limit who could be covered for breast reduction surgery. He also stated that a range of criteria be used to assess whether a breast reduction was medically required, not just the weight of the breast tissue.

As someone who struggles with her weight, I just love Dr Schnur for saying this:

"The overweight woman who presents for a mammoplasty raises another question. Third-party payers often state that if the patient would lose weight, her symptoms would improve and therefore, this is the preferred treatment. While this may be true, if a woman cannot lose weight, why hold her hostage because of her weight problem?"

Every woman responds differently to the physical symptoms of having large breasts. I believe that breast reduction should be considered within the context of an individual woman's life. Medical literature has proven just how much breast reduction surgery improves the quality of a woman's life – regardless of the weight of breast tissue removed.

Weight Not Volume

Unfortunately, insurers don't take into account breast volume, only weight. If you think of a breast as a pillow, some pillows are dense, they don't compact, and they weigh a lot. Other pillows are large, condense a lot, and don't weigh much at all. It's like a small heavy foam pillow compared to a large light feather pillow. Insurance providers focus on weight, not cup size. Unfortunately, liposuctioned fat cannot be applied to the weight total.

Document & Get Evidence

Most insurers will require your surgeon to provide a letter describing your symptoms and physical findings, estimating the breast weight to be removed, and requesting coverage.

This must be done before you schedule your surgery. Your insurer may not be obligated to pay for the surgery if it was not pre-authorized!

Make sure you document and get evidence to support your claim, such as from other doctors, physiotherapists, chiropractors, etc. to show that your breast reduction surgery is required medically.

If your insurer denies covering you because they have assessed your surgery as being cosmetic, ask your surgeon to educate the insurer about symptomatic macromastia (symptoms of large breasts) and to explain the difference between breast reduction and breast lift (which is cosmetic).

For Australians, if you can get some of your costs covered by your health insurance, make sure you have a good referral from your doctor stating that you are having the breast reduction for medical reasons (back, neck and shoulder pain and headaches are common medical reasons). Medicare may also give you a rebate on different "item numbers" from your surgery. So, keep all your receipts and put in a claim.

Appeal

If your insurer denies covering your surgery (and you know breast reduction is necessary for your health and well-being), you are legally entitled to appeal the decision. The appeal process is normally described in your denial letter. There may be multiple levels of appeal available to you.

In your appeal, include a letter describing your symptoms and how they affect or limit your life (focus on real physical issues rather than say fashion issues). Also provide letters from a family doctor, orthopedist, physical therapist, chiropractor, or massage therapist to support your appeal. Your surgeon can also submit a personal letter, stating up-to-date scientific information and medical literature to support treatment of symptomatic macromastia.

Teaching Hospital

If you don't have health insurance or your insurer won't cover breast reduction, and you don't have the money to pay for it yourself, you could try a plastic surgery clinic in a teaching hospital. Residents can do your surgery under supervision and the cost is minimal. In New York for example, residents are trained at Lenox Hill Hospital and apparently do good work.

Overseas Surgery Options

Many women living in the US, UK, Canada, New Zealand and Australia, are choosing to have their breast reduction surgery in places like Thailand. You may have seen some TV shows about this. Women fly into Bangkok, for example, and are taken to a luxury hotel. They then have an appointment with their surgeon and a day or so later, they come back and have their surgery. After surgery, they stay at their hotel again.

If cost is an issue, you may find that this is a cheaper alternative. But do your research and choose your surgeon wisely. You want someone who is experienced and highly qualified.

My Experience

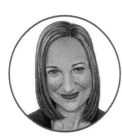

Ayesha: After 15 years as a loyal customer of my health insurance provider, I was shocked that none of my surgery costs were covered. A friend who had her health insurance with a different provider got her hospital stay covered by her insurance which saved her more than $4,000.

Here's an itemized list of the cost of my surgery (in Australian dollars):

- Initial Consultation with Surgeon: **$250**
  (If you are interviewing three surgeons to find the best one for you, you can times this by three.)

- Surgeon's Fee: **$8,000**

- Theatre & Accommodation: **$3,700**

- Anesthesia Fees: **$2,200**

- Prescription Medication: **$30**

- Post-Surgery Bras: **$90**

Total Cost: $14,270

On top of this, I had to add in transport costs as I flew interstate to have my surgery. I did get a rebate of about $1,200 from Medicare (Australia's public health system).

When I went to the first surgeon, a general surgeon and not a cosmetic or plastic surgeon, her quote was under $5,000. But she would only do a breast lift.

I went to a private clinic where I felt like I would get the best surgery and care. It cost me a lot more than going to a public hospital, but I felt like the cost was worth it. But it was a huge expense.

When I had first arranged my surgery, I was under the impression that it would only cost me $8,000 out of pocket, but I later found out that my health insurance wouldn't cover a single cent.

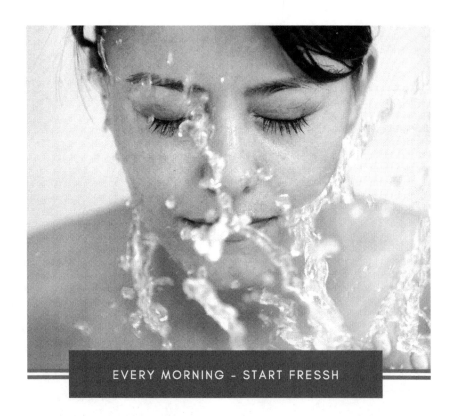

EVERY MORNING - START FRESSH

Today is a new day

HOW WILL YOU CARE FOR YOURSELF TODAY?

56

CHAPTER 11

Post-Op Breast Size

You probably have some idea what breast size you would like to have after your breast reduction. Unfortunately, there is no way to guarantee what size your breasts will end up being.

It really depends on what happens during your surgery, which is determined by your individual anatomy, how much skin and tissue need to be removed, and the type of surgery technique the surgeon is using as well as the blood flow to the tissue while you are in surgery.

You can, however, discuss your ideal breast size with your surgeon who will be able to give you a good indication of what the outcome will be.

You may feel stressed about choosing a breast size. At the end of the day, only you can determine what is right for you. If you've had a lot of back and neck pain for many years due to your breasts, you will want your breasts to be small enough to reduce your physical symptoms while still feeling like yourself. It can be a shock for some to go from having ample cleavage to none in some cases.

Size Considerations

Consider the following when you are choosing a post-op breast size:

- **Are you going to be having any more children?**
  Often your breast will increase in size during pregnancy and breastfeeding. Think about what size your breasts

might be in the future if you do have more children. If you want to breastfeed in the future, you need to discuss this with your surgeon because maintaining breast functionality can impact the type of surgery you have.

- **Gravity & Aging**
  Alas, gravity does play a role in boob droop. Consider what time and aging will do to the post-op size of your boobs.

- **Hormonal Changes**
  Hormones can impact the size of your breasts. Changes in hormones can be caused by pregnancy, menopause, birth control pills and hormonal issues. Any of these can impact the size of your breasts after surgery.

- **Think Volume Not Cup Size**
  You've probably bought a bra that's your normal size and found that it is either too big or too small. There's a lack of consistency in bra sizing. You may want to think of volume when considering your desired breast size. You can use a bag of rice, for example, to show the volume you're keen on.

- **In-Between Sizes**
  Many women ask for a large B or a small C for their reduction. The problem with this is that bras come in B or C, not small C or big B. You won't want to have the problem of bursting out of a B cup and swimming in a C cup. Standard sizing is best if your surgeon can achieve it depending on what happens during the surgery.

- **Body Proportions**
  You do not have to get breasts that are in proportion to your body size. However, you may like to think about how you will look with different size breasts in proportion to the rest of you.

- **Your Desire**
  Only you can say what is truly right for you. I didn't want to go to a very small A or B cup. I was happy with a C cup. A friend really wanted to be an A to B cup. She did

what was right for her, and she's happy. I did what was
right for me, and I'm happy too.

Getting Real

Once you have an idea of what size you'd like your breasts
to be, you need to discuss this with your surgeon. Talking to
your surgeon about your expectations is vital to your satisfaction after your surgery. Your surgeon should listen to your
request and give appropriate advice about what is possible
and what is not.

Breast surgery, unlike other aesthetic surgery such as a nose
job, is not as predictable. This is because the anatomy of
your breasts plays a big role what is possible during surgery.
One of the key things during breast reduction surgery is
ensuring the nipples survive. Sometimes going too small can
jeopardize the nipple. Issues can become evident during the
surgery that may mean the surgeon has to modify their approach based on what is happening at the time.

During surgery, the flap (pedicle) remains attached to the
nipple to contain both arteries and veins. Nipples require a
blood supply to survive and can die due to lack of inflow from
the arteries or lack of outflow from veins. A surgeon might
have to decide during the surgery to save your nipples over
making your breasts even smaller. If the surgeon doesn't do
this, then a patient could lose their nipples.

The key thing during surgery is for the nipples to survive.
If there is a problem during surgery, nipple survival will be
more important than size. And I for one would prefer to have
larger breasts and functioning nipples.

Discuss with Your Surgeon

When you have your initial consult with the surgeon, ask
them what size they would recommend. Also, give them your
preference.

If you have a plastic surgeon that is not interested in your input about size, you need to ask them why. They may have a good reason. You don't want to be bullied into a size that you don't want. But if you understand what is possible, and what isn't, then it is easier to make a decision about going ahead with surgery.

This is why it is also important to consult with more than one surgeon. You will get a feel for who you prefer, their respect for your wishes, and how they explain information about the surgery. A good surgeon will take time to listen to what you want and take your preferences into account.

Please note, you won't know what your new breast size is until sometime after your surgery. You will have a lot of swelling for some time, and it can take up to six to 12 months to see your true size.

Arlene's Story

I had waited for years to have a breast reduction. It was a dream come true. I had saved up $10,000. I'd found a great surgeon. And I was ready to start living a new life with smaller breasts.

My surgery seemed to go well. I was sent home the day after surgery with no complications. A few days later, I started to have problems. I rang my surgeon's office and told them that the incision going from the nipple down to the bottom of the breast had started to open on both breasts. I was freaking out.

My surgeon told me to come straight in. One of the nurses on his team checked me out. She put some antiseptic cream on them and covered them with tape. She told me that that a wound breakdown was common after breast reduction, though having both breasts with a wound breakdown wasn't as common. Though the nurse was helpful, I was still nervous when I went home. I would have liked to have seen the surgeon, but he was in surgery.

I didn't know how long it would take for the wound to heal normally. I kept applying the antiseptic cream the nurse had given me. The next week the wounds were still open, so I had an appointment with the surgeon. He told me it would take some time for the wound to heal. He gave me instructions on how to best help my breasts heal.

I've got to say, it was stressful. I didn't even know that wound breakdown was a possibility. I used to cry when I looked in the mirror. I could see parts of my breast I didn't know existed. It was quite gross. Eventually, the wounds did heal, but it took a long time. I have a larger scar down the front of my breasts that I had expected. Even though I had all these problems with my scars healing, 12 months later, I am relieved to have smaller breasts.

CHAPTER 12

Breastfeeding After a Reduction

While many women choose to wait until they've finished having children and breastfeeding before having a reduction, for others, this isn't an option.

Other women may not have met someone they would like to have children with and wonder if they ever will. They don't want to put off having their breast reduction for a scenario that may or may not eventuate.

Some women have a breast reduction without considering the impact it will have on future breastfeeding. For others, it just feels too abstract and irrelevant for where they are in their life at the time of surgery.

No doubt, you have your own story about why you want to have breast reduction and whether you want to breastfeed in the future.

I think it is important for women to make informed choices about their bodies that will support their wishes now but also in the long-term.

Right now, a baby may be the furthest thing from your mind, especially if you're really young. However, I want you to have the knowledge you need to make an empowered decision that suits where you are now in your life, and that keeps your options open.

Why Breastfeeding is Important

I am a big advocate for breastfeeding; I breastfed for about five years in total. Breastfeeding was important to me, and I didn't want to risk my ability to breastfeed by having my breast reduction surgery until after I'd finished having children.

That said, I don't believe breastfeeding is always best when a mother and baby are not thriving. There are situations where breastfeeding needs to be supplemented or abandoned altogether. At the end of the day, the most important thing is the well-being of the mother and child.

There are a number of advantages to breastfeeding for both the baby and mother.

Benefits of Breastfeeding for the Baby

- Breastfeeding is convenient, free, and always on hand

- Breast milk is specially formulated for your baby and adapts to their needs

- Breast milk contains antibodies that help your baby fight off viruses and bacteria

- Breastfed babies normally have less gas and constipation

- Breastfed babies normally have higher IQs

- Breastfeeding lowers your baby's risk of having asthma or allergies

- Babies who are breastfed exclusively for the first six months without any formula, have fewer ear infections, respiratory illnesses, and bouts of diarrhea

- Breastfed babies tend to have few cavities

- Breastfed babies benefit from being held more

- Breastfeeding promotes healthy mother-baby bonding

- Breastfeeding halves the risk of Sudden Infant Death Syndrome (SIDS)

- Over the course of their lifetime, breastfed babies have a decreased risk of malnutrition, obesity and heart disease compared to formula fed babies

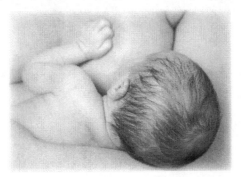

Benefits of Breastfeeding for the Mother

- Better healing after delivery, as baby's sucking causes the mother's uterus to contract and reduces the flow of blood after delivery

- Breastfeeding can help a woman lose weight gained during pregnancy

- Mothers that breastfeed are less likely to develop breast cancer later in life

- A vacation from menstruation while lactating

- Breast feeding is more economical than bottle feeding

- Breastfeeding promotes healthy mother-baby bonding

- During breastfeeding, hormones are released, creating feelings of calm and warmth in the mother

"It is also important to remember that nursing is so much more than nutrition. By breastfeeding our babies, we meet a whole range of emotional needs as well. When we understand success in this way, we are aware of the power we have to make breastfeeding possible and to be wholly satisfied with whatever unique direction our breastfeeding relationship may take. It is this empowerment that gives us strength in vulnerable moments and keeps the knowledge uppermost in our minds that we alone determine what success will mean for us."
Diana West

How Breast Reduction Affects Breast Feeding

The aim of breast reduction is to reduce the quantity of breast tissue. When this tissue is removed, milk ducts and glandular tissue are also removed, and can, therefore, impact whether breast milk can be produced. Many women, however, do successfully breastfeed after a reduction.

The type of surgery you have, along with any complications, will have a big impact on whether breastfeeding post-reduction is possible.

If you have a **free nipple graft** (FNG), you will not be able to breastfeed because it involves totally removing the nipple and areola. This is why a free nipple graft should be avoided if possible if you want to breastfeed. If for some reason, this is the only option available to you, you really want to breastfeed in the future, you may consider postponing your surgery until you have had children.

While a **liposuction-only** reduction does not normally affect breastfeeding, it only removes a limited amount of breast tissue and does not provide any lift to the breasts.

Pedicle surgical methods, such as the Vertical/Anchor or the Inverted-T/Lollipop, give you a high chance of breastfeeding because the areola and nipple function are normally maintained.

66

It is important to note that if you have your **areola resized**, there is a greater risk of damaging the nerves that are part of the letdown reflex (this is the reflex that tells your body to release milk).

The letdown reflex is important because it allows milk to be produced and stored in your breasts, ready for when your baby needs to feed. If your letdown reflex is affected or doesn't occur, less milk gets removed from your breasts which can then impact your milk supply.

If you let your surgeon know you want to breastfeed when you have children, they can make sure enough of the areola complex remains in order to maximize your ability to breast-feed in the future.

There are no guarantees that just because you have a pedicle type of breast reduction, that you will be able to breastfeed. The truth is, you won't know until you're holding your sweet baby in your arms.

How Breastfeeding Affect Breast Size

Many women experience a change in the breasts during pregnancy as their body prepares for breastfeeding. Breasts will get bigger during pregnancy and may return to the size they were before you had surgery. This can be a scary prospect for many women, however, keep in mind that pregnancy increases breast size, not lactation. With or without surgery, your breasts are likely to increase during pregnancy. After the birth of your baby and the first few weeks of breastfeeding, your breasts should return to their pre-pregnancy size. If your breasts enlarge a lot during pregnancy, you may find you have more stretch marks afterwards.

Maximizing Milk Supply

Some women, whether they have had a breast reduction or not, experience milk supply issues. Women who have had a breast reduction often have a higher chance of having low milk supply. However, this doesn't mean you can't breast-feed. There are things you can do to try and increase your supply. And if necessary, you supplement breastfeeding with formula.

Things that affect milk supply include stress, medications, positioning and attachment of baby to the breast, diet and hydration.

To maximize your breast milk supply:

• Consider **natural pain relief** options during labor if possible.

• Have **skin-to-skin contact** with your baby as soon as you can after birth (even if you have a caesarean) – this not only helps you bond with your baby, it also impacts the hormones that help your milk come in.

• **Room-in** with your baby, being in close proximity to your baby will likewise help with bonding and hormones, as well as enabling you to respond to your baby's needs quickly.

• Understand that breastfeeding is a **skill -** many women think they and their baby should know how to breastfeed, but for most women, this isn't true.

• Make sure your baby is **attaching** to the breast properly – poor attachment leads to bleeding and painful nipples.

• Stay **hydrated** – your body needs hydration to be able to create milk.

• **Get support** – get advice and support from your midwife, lactation consultant, or doctor.

• Try to **relax** and enjoy motherhood (even if you don't know what you're doing most of the time).

• **Avoid supplementing** with formula if possible, if your

baby is distressed and hungry, you may need to give them formula (just be aware that your milk supply can diminish if your baby doesn't feed enough from your breast, creating further supply issues).

- **Supplement** in ways that are supportive of breastfeeding. If you are supplementing with formula, you could try a **Supplemental Feeding System.** This is a feeding tube device that mimics breastfeeding (the advantage of this over a bottle is that the baby is less likely to develop breast refusal – which is where the baby prefers the ease of a bottle over the work of milking the breast, leading to refusing the breast).

- You may need to try **medication** to increase your milk supply – some medical conditions can impact milk supply (such as diabetes or Polycystic Ovary Syndrome, your doctor can prescribe medication that can increase your milk supply).

- Try eating **foods** that may help with milk supply including oatmeal, salmon, spinach and beet leaves, carrots, fennel seeds, fenugreek seeds, garlic, sesame seeds, alfalfa and basil leaves.

- Drink **teas** that may help increase your milk supply, such as special lactation teas (you would probably have to order these online), red raspberry leaf, alfalfa, fenugreek, black tea, anise seed, blessed thistle, and marshmallow root.

Define Your Own Success

We live in a world of constant judgment. As a new mother, you will undoubtedly receive advice from people with good intentions who only want what is best for you and your baby. Their advice will depend on their view of the world. Some will tell you to give up on breastfeeding because it's too hard, especially if you have supply issues. Others may tell you your baby needs breast milk or they will be scarred for life. Breast reduction surgery often brings out a lot of judgment as well!

As women, we need to define our own success. If breastfeeding is important to you, then do it in whatever way works best for you.

Here's a quote from the book, Defining Your Own Success: Breastfeeding After Breast Reduction Surgery by Diana West:

"Among women who have had breast reduction surgery and are now breastfeeding, it is often said that "We each define our own success." As it is used here, "success" is not an absolute term referring to a continuum of less to more milk produced. Rather, it is defined by the degree of satisfaction each woman and her baby derive from the breastfeeding relationship they create together. It is not determined by the amount of milk a woman produces. Each woman's experience of success will be different; some may be able to breastfeed exclusively, while others may need to supplement the baby's entire nutritional requirement."

My wish for you, and all mothers, is that you do what is right for you and your baby, and that you get the support you need.

Get More Information

Breastfeeding after a reduction is a big topic. To explore this issue more, you may like to check out these books:

- **Defining Your Own Success: Breastfeeding after Breast Reduction Surgery** by Diana West

- **Breastfeeding after Breast and Nipple Procedures** by Diana West and Elliot Hirsch

- **The Breastfeeding Mother's Guide to Making More Milk** by Diana West and Lisa Marasco

For more information on these books and on breastfeeding after a reduction, you may like to visit the Breast Feeding After Reduction website: www.bfar.org

70

CHAPTER 13

Find Surgeon

Once you've decided to have a breast reduction, the most important decision you have to make is choosing your surgeon. If you are undecided, meeting with a surgeon should help you with your decision.

Consider the process of choosing a surgeon like you're interviewing them for a job – the most important role of transforming your large boobs into smaller breasts.

Find a Surgeon

Tracking down a good surgeon can feel like hard work. You can start with your general practitioner or primary care doctor as they will be writing your referral anyway.

When considering a surgeon, you want a doctor that is board-certified. Choosing a board-certified plastic surgeon means you can be sure that the doctor has graduated from an accredited medical school.

To find a surgeon, you can look at various websites/organizations including:

- American Society of Plastic Surgeons (ASAPS)
  www.plasticsurgery.org

- Australian Society of Plastic Surgeons (ASPS)
  www.plasticsurgery.org.au

- British Association of Aesthetic Plastic Surgeons (BAAPS)
  www.baaps.org.uk

- New Zealand Association of Plastic Surgeons (NZAPS)
  www.plasticsurgery.org.nz

Referral from Your General Practitioner/Primary Doctor

You will most likely require a referral from your primary care doctor. Your doctor should have no problems writing you a referral. In Australia, you can use your referral with any surgeon even if it has another surgeon's details on it. So, you can either get your doctor to do multiple referrals to the different surgeons you are considering, or you can take copies of the referral and use the same one.

I suggest keeping a copy for your own records regardless. My referral went missing and was important for me to get a rebate for Medicare. I had to get my primary doctor to re-issue the referral just days before my surgery.

What to Look for in a Surgeon

When choosing a surgeon, you need to focus on the following:

- **Rapport**
  Do you feel comfortable with the surgeon? Do you feel like you can ask them questions?

- **Qualifications/Accreditation**
  Do they have the appropriate qualifications and accreditation?

- **Inclusions**
  What is included in the costs of the surgery? What happens if there is a complication?

- **Surgery Location**
  Where will the surgery happen? Hospital? Day surgery

72

clinic?

- **Answers to Interview Questions**
  The way the surgeon responds to your questions will give you a good idea about whether they are right for you.

Evaluate your surgeon as well as their practice. If the office staff are rude, impatient or unhelpful, that's not a good sign. You want to feel as comfortable as possible during the breast reduction process.

I strongly recommended you have consults three different surgeons. This will give you a good perspective and help you choose the right surgeon.

Initial Consultation

Once you have found a surgeon you would like to meet with, you will schedule an initial consult. In this appointment, the surgeon will measure and evaluate your breasts. You will need to take off your top and bra. The surgeon will most likely lift your breasts and physically examine them.

If you are uncomfortable about this, take a support person with you (such as a partner, friend or relative with whom you are comfortable about seeing your breasts). You can also ask for a nurse to be present with you during the consultation.

The surgeon may take photos of your breasts at this time or at a later consult.

They will discuss your breast reduction options with you.

Organize Your Documents

During the breast reduction process, you will acquire a lot of paper! You want to be organized so that you can quickly find what you need. I recommend having a file for all your relevant documents.

Here are some of the things you will need to put in your file:

- Information and brochures provided by surgeons

- Quotes from surgeons

- Contract for your surgery

- Insurance documents and claim forms

- All medical receipts

- Any other relevant documents

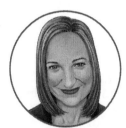

Ayesha: My GP referred me to a local surgeon. My then husband and I met with her. At the time, we didn't realize that she was a general surgeon and not a cosmetic surgeon. She showed us her portfolio of breast surgeries. I would rather keep my massive drooping boobs than end up like one of her patients. As we talked with the surgeon, she said that she would only do a lift for me and not a reduction. I'm glad I didn't choose her as my surgeon. I ended up going with a surgeon in another state that a friend has used. I knew that this surgeon was highly skilled and could do the reduction I needed.

Anita's Story

I'm a midwife. I'm on my feet all day caring for women and their babies. By the end of a shift, my back and neck are so sore. I wear an E cup bra, and my shoulders have large indents in them from the bra strap digging into me. As I've gotten older, I've noticed that my back and neck are getting worse.

I spoke to my doctor and chiropractor about it and they both suggested I have a breast reduction. I wasn't sure at first, but the more I thought about it, the more I liked the idea.

I've done a lot of research, and I met with three different surgeons. I finally settled on one that is a few hours' drive away. I had a good rapport with her and feel like she is the best surgeon for me.

I'm scheduled to have surgery in two months. I'm so excited. As a medical professional, I know there are risks with any surgery, but thankfully, breast reduction has fewer risks that most surgery. I'm hoping to go down to a B or C cup.

Happiness is not something
you postpone for the
future; it is something you
design for the present.

JIM ROHN

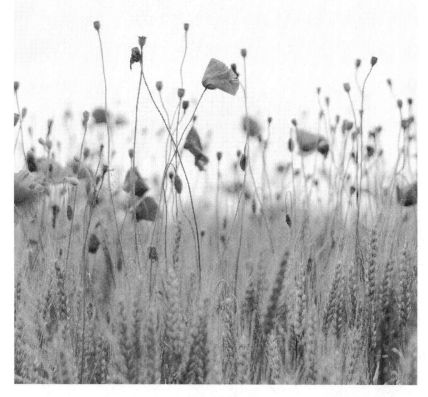

CHAPTER 14

Questions to Ask Your Surgeon

It is important that you get as much information as possible from your prospective surgeon. As you will see below, there are a lot of things to ask your surgeon. I wish I had a copy of this list before my surgery!

Asking these questions does several things:

- It lets the plastic surgeon know that you are informed, and that you are taking the surgery seriously.

- It helps you get to know if the surgeon has integrity and if they will stand by you if there is a complication.

- It helps you choose the right surgeon for you.

- It gives you peace of mind once you have chosen a surgeon who has integrity, and will take care of you if something did go wrong.

Key Questions

Here are key questions to ask your surgeon about:

1. The surgeon's experience and **qualifications**

2. Breast reduction **risks**

3. How they manage **problems** if they arise

77

4. Whether you qualify for **insurance** coverage

5. The surgeon's **surgical preference** and what you can expect from the surgery

6. Information on **recovery** after surgery

1 Surgeon's Experience & Qualifications

- Are you board certified?

- How many years have you been performing breast reduction surgery? Approximately how many breast reductions have you done in your career thus far?

- How many breast reductions do you perform per week? (You want a surgeon who does breast reductions regularly.)

- Are you a cosmetic/plastic surgeon or a general surgeon? (Trust me, you want a cosmetic surgeon, not a general surgeon.)

- Do you have any before and after pictures to show me? If not, why? (I would be hesitant to go with a surgeon who does not show you a portfolio of their work.)

2 Breast Reduction Risks

- What are the three worst things that can happen after this surgery?

- What are the chances of each of those happening?

- What do we do if those things happen?

- What are some of the complications that some of your past patients have encountered?

3. Managing Problems

- What if something goes wrong – what happens then? (Will they help you or leave you in the lurch?)

- What if I am not happy with the size of my breasts after surgery (if they are smaller or bigger than we agreed upon)? Or if I am still in back pain because they are still too big? What then?

- What if I have a problem that is not your fault or I have healing problems that are unique to me and not due to something you did? How is that handled?

- What if I develop a scarring problem and need a scar revision? What will you do?

- What are dog ears, and what will you do to resolve them if I get them? Is this covered in the cost or will this be an additional cost?

- How do you treat keloid or hypertrophic scarring if it occurs?

4. Insurance

- Will my insurance cover the cost of surgery? Will there be any out-of-pocket expenses?

- If I require additional procedures (corrective), are they also covered by insurance?

- What is the process for getting my insurance to pay for this surgery?

5. About Your Particular Surgery

- What is the procedure you would use on me, and why?

- What determines whether I have a free nipple graft?

- If I meet the criteria for a free nipple graft, would you try to do the inferior pedicle first and then proceed with the free nipple graft if it doesn't work?

- Will there be ANY sensation left if I do have a free nipple graft?

- If you do the breast reduction in accordance with the proportions of my body, what do you see as "in proportion" to the rest of my body? (Ask for an approximate size such as between a B and a C?)

- Do I get any say in what size my breasts will be?

- As proportion is subjective, is it my right to choose a size that is different from what you think looks good?

- Can you guesstimate the gram removal?

- Does the tissue get sent to the lab after removal for analysis? (Good surgeons will send your tissue off for analysis.)

- Can you tell me approximately how long the surgery will be?

- How do you determine the size of the nipple/areola complex? Can I have any say in the size of my new areolas?

- Do you prefer to use drains? If so, when will the drains be removed?

- Where will the surgery be performed?

- Will I stay overnight?

- Will I have the opportunity to meet the anesthesiologist before my surgery?

- What pain medications will I be given?

- Can I discuss anti-nausea medications and concerns with the anesthesiologist?

- What if I get a cold before my surgery?

- Do I continue to take my regular medications before surgery?

- What medications do I avoid before surgery and immediately after surgery?

- Do I require any special tests before surgery?

- Do you have someone who assists you in surgery?

- Does he/she work on one breast while you work on the other?

- Will I end up with two entirely different looking breasts if I have two surgeons?

- When do you do the markings for surgery?

- Do I need to pre-book extra appointments?

- Do you insert a catheter during surgery?

- Will I have a tube put down my throat?

6. **Recovery**

- How much time do I need to take off work?

- How long until I can resume normal exercise and activity?

- How long until I can drive?

- When can I resume my normal sex life?

- How long after surgery will it be before the breasts drop into a nice shape?

81

A professional surgeon will be happy to answer these questions. So please do not be afraid to ask these questions and any others you think of. I suggest you take a list of questions to your initial consultation with the surgeon (or take this book!). You won't remember all the questions you want to ask, so it is better to be prepared.

It can be challenging to contemplate something going wrong, but you need to be as informed as possible, and choose a surgeon that is going to take care of you if something did go wrong. You don't want to put yourself in the position of dealing with a complication without the full support of your surgeon.

This is your body and you need to be assertive about your needs, wants, and expectations. Surgeons are not gods. They are mortals skilled with a scalpel. You have a duty to yourself to make sure you are getting the best surgeon for you. And remember, you are the client – the surgeon works for you!

Plastic Surgeon Preferences

Surgeons have different preferences that they have developed and used during the course of their training and practice. These preferences may play a role in whether you choose a particular surgeon or not. You can ask the surgeon about their preferences as your initial consult.

Inpatient/Outpatient

Many surgeons do breast reductions on an outpatient basis. This means that you enter and leave hospital the same day. Unless there are complications, you will not have the option to stay longer. You also need to check with your insurance provider about whether they will cover you if you do need to stay in hospital overnight.

I believe that staying overnight is preferable because this is major surgery. You want medical attention if something goes wrong. Also, it is good to have pain relief and fluids administered via an IV. Most women say that staying overnight was a good thing for their recovery because they felt more comfortable knowing they were being cared for by professional medical staff.

Of course, there are others who find it more restful to return to their own bed and home. Being in a hospital environment does come with a lot of noise and interruptions.

Hospital vs. Surgical Clinic

Most breast reductions are performed in hospitals. However, there are some surgeons who perform their surgeries in a surgical clinic or center. If the surgeon operates in a clinic or center, please find out how well equipped they are to deal with emergencies since they are not a proper hospital.

Check the following:

- Find out what the procedure is if there is an emergency or complication during surgery

- Make sure the surgical clinic is fully accredited in your country

- Make sure the anesthesiologists are board-certified medical doctors

If the surgical clinic and staff are fully accredited, then it is no more dangerous to have your surgery there than at a hospital. The surgical team will be trained in the same way as hospital staff and will have good equipment on site to deal with emergencies.

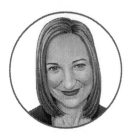

Ayesha: There are pros and cons with both environments. I was initially scheduled to have my surgery in a public hospital in my hometown. I wasn't happy with the surgeon's skills and opted to have the surgery in a private clinic in another city. This clinic was fairly new, state of the art, with exceptional facilities and staff. I felt safer going to the clinic that I did to the hospital. It is a personal choice that only you can make. And the food was delicious (though I wasn't in a state to appreciate it).

Drains/No Drains

The use of drains varies by surgeon and can be a topical issue. Apparently, drains help significantly with the amount of post-op swelling. Drains are often left in for about 24 hours, but in some cases up to a week.

As a patient, you probably won't have any say about whether you have drains or not. It will be part of the surgeon's procedures – they either use drains or they don't. If you have strong feelings either way, please discuss these with your surgeon.

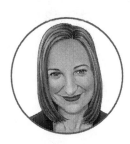

Ayesha: I had drains as part of my surgery. I cannot say whether I healed better because of them or not. I still had a fair amount of post-op swelling. They do leave small scars. I didn't even know about drains until I woke up with one in each side

Stitches/Staples/Glue

The method of "sewing" you up after your surgery will depend on the surgeon's personal and professional preference.

Staples: these can lead to the most scarring, especially if left in too long. Many surgeons have moved away from staples, and it is no longer a favored method of closing an incision. Sometimes a surgeon may use a couple of temporary staples to hold things together while they are suturing the incision. They then remove the staples straight away.

Glues: are used either by themselves or with other suture methods. Some people are highly allergic to the glue but don't know until it is too late. If your surgeon plans to use glue, I suggest you do a patch test before your surgery. You don't want to have a severe allergic reaction over your recovering wound.

Stitches: these are the most common form of closing the incisions. Often, surgeons will use dissolving sutures to close the wounds. Many surgeons now use some clear, colorless sutures which disintegrate slowly (often taking six months post-op to dissolve). Sometimes women experience a suture knot coming up to the surface and needs to be removed by the surgeon. If your surgeon doesn't use dissolving sutures, you will need to have them removed by the surgeon or one of their staff.

Marita's Story

I recently had breast reduction surgery. I'm turning 66 next month. It's funny to think about having a cosmetic style of surgery at this age for my breasts. I'm a widow and mother of two. My husband died of a heart attack five years ago. He was definitely a breast man and he loved my large bosom. All my life, I took care of my husband and children, and never did much for myself. As one my friends often says, I ate the cold toast and the smallest chop.

Many years after my husband died, I went on a few dates. I was very conscious of my breasts. I wished they were smaller. It was affecting my confidence. Not only were they large and heavy, they were also pendulous. The skin on my chest was very fine, and I had a lot of stretch marks. In my youth I had accepted that I had big breasts, and there was nothing I could do about it.

The idea to get a breast reduction came from a TV show I saw about a plastic surgeon in Thailand. One woman had a facelift, one a breast enlargement, and the other a breast reduction. Honestly, up until that moment in time, I'd ever considered any cosmetic surgery, let alone a breast reduction.

Every few weeks, I would start thinking about breast reduction. The idea would pop into my head at the strangest of times. Eventually, I spoke to my doctor about it. She was very supportive and referred me to a local surgeon. I was worried that I would be too old to have surgery and that I was foolish wanting to have a reduction at my age.

However, I met with the surgeon who assured me that I was a good candidate for a reduction as I was in good health and that I had a fair amount of breast tissue to remove. Before I knew it, I'd made my decision, and was booked in for my surgery.

I told my son and daughter that I was having surgery and they were shocked initially but ended up being very supportive. I stayed with my son and his wife after the surgery, and they took good care of me.

My body responded to the surgery well despite my age. I was out of it for about ten days. I was tired, a little moody, and in some discomfort. My breasts are healing well.

Last week, I was shopping for new bras, and I had tears in my eyes as I thought, "Why hadn't I done this sooner."

My breast reduction, though late in life, has given me a new lease on life!

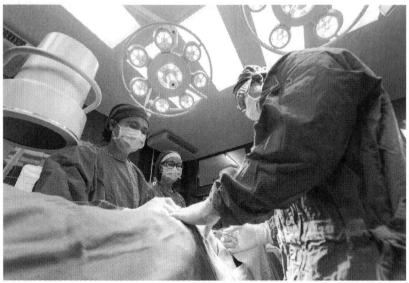

"I did that many years ago [breast reduction], because at five-foot-one, I had boobs like Dolly Parton. I've never thought big boobs were good. I hated them the second I got them. I did nothing but try to hide them my whole life, and as soon as I was in college I was like, 'These have got to go' ... When I did stand-up, people would heckle me because such a short person with such big boobs is very distracting."

Janeane Garofalo
Actress, comedian and activist, – Inked Magazine

CHAPTER 15

Make Your Decision

Are you ready to make a decision about breast reduction surgery? Have you already made up your mind? Or, are you still undecided?

By now, you've probably done a fair bit of research. You have hopefully read this book up to this point. And hopefully, you have been able to talk to your friends and family about what you're thinking.

If you're still not sure, the best thing to do is to meet with at least one surgeon, if you haven't already. They can give you a really good idea about what you can expect after they have assessed your breasts.

Here are some things to consider in your decision-making process:

- **Benefits**
  What benefits will you get from having breast reduction surgery?

- **Risks**
  Are you willing to take the risk of complications of surgery?

- **Scarring**
  Are you comfortable will having scars on your breasts?

- **Recovery Time**
  Can you have enough time off work and home duties to allow yourself to recover? Do you have support to help

you during the recovery?

- **Breast Size**
  Are you going to go down enough in size to get the benefits of a smaller bust and make it worth the cost and discomfort?

- **Cost**
  Do you have the money to have surgery?

- **Insurance**
  Will your insurance provider cover any of the costs?

This is a life-changing and expensive decision; one that you do not want to take lightly. This is your body and it is your choice. Trust your instincts. If you have a bad feeling about a surgeon, no matter how highly regarded they are, go with your gut. Feel into what is right for you.

Demi's Story

I went up a cup size every year in high school. When I graduated, I was wearing an H cup. I'm small framed, so I looked really out of proportion. Throughout my 20s, I struggled with back and neck pain. I also struggled to find clothes to fit properly. To fit my boobs, I'd have to wear a tent-like top or dress.

When I would visit my GP, I would mention my back pain. I had a plan, you see, to get breast reduction surgery eventually, and I wanted to have it documented that I had ongoing back and neck pain.

Eventually, my GP gave me a referral to a local plastic surgeon. I was so excited to go and meet them. I had a ton of questions prepared. I'm an A-type personality, and I had scoured the internet to find out everything I could before my

90

appointment. I loved my surgeon straight away and knew she was the one I wanted to do the surgery. Because I had a long history of back and neck pain, as well as a ton of breast tissue to be removed, my insurance provider agreed to cover the surgery.

I scheduled my surgery around my husband's holidays, so he could help me with our three young children. When the big day arrived, I was so excited. Finally, after all these years of waiting, I was going to have my dream come true.

The surgery went well. I had to be careful with the kids. They would want to jump all over me, and they accidentally hurt me a few times. I had my surgery six months ago. My breasts have settled down; they were very swollen for a long time. I love my new breasts! I feel like I am more in proportion and shopping is so much fun now. I've got a whole new wardrobe. No more tent dresses for me.

"They were like French bread. They're round, not oblong now. [Now] when I [lie] down they don't cover my nose."
Patricia Heaton, Actress,
Star of Everyone Loves Raymond – People Magazine

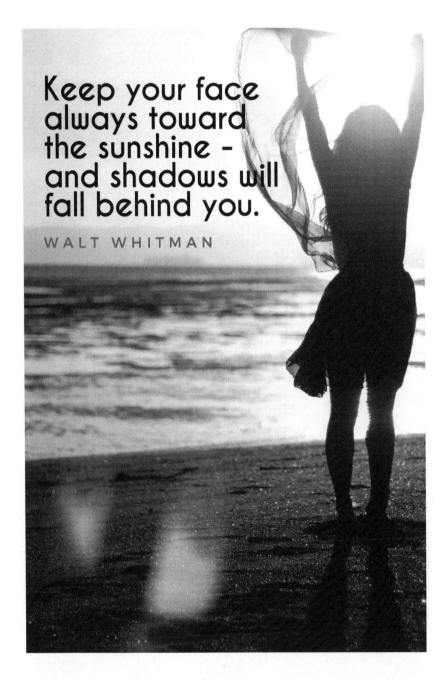

Keep your face always toward the sunshine - and shadows will fall behind you.

WALT WHITMAN

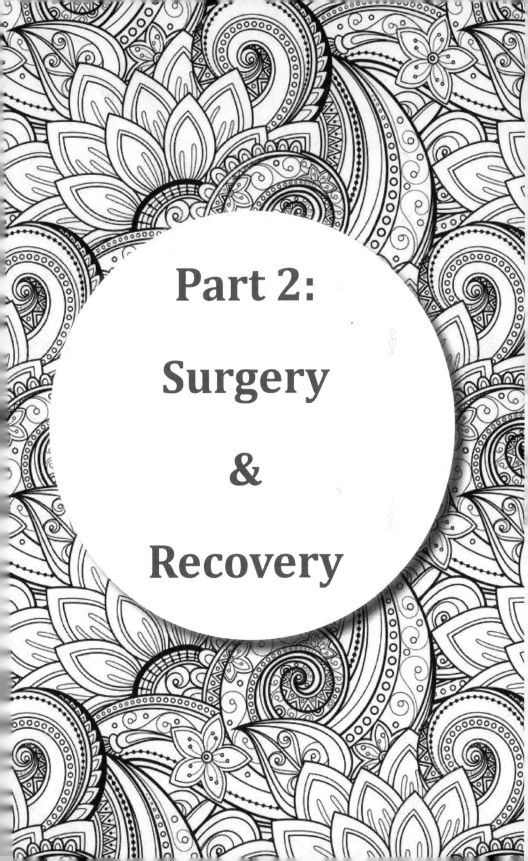

Part 2:

Surgery

&

Recovery

Part 2: Surgery & Recovery

Welcome to Part 2 where you will find
out about your surgery, including:

- How to prepare for surgery

- What to expect on the day of your surgery

- What to expect during your recovery

- Understand what your breast may be like after surgery

- How to minimize scar tissue

- Manage itching and burning

- What to eat to maximize your recovery

- Be prepared for post-op blues

- And tips for caring for young children after surgery

CHAPTER 16

Preparing for Surgery

You've made a decision to go ahead with breast reduction surgery. You have found a surgeon you trust. You've organized your insurance (if they will cover you). And you're got your surgery date! You are probably excited and possibly a bit scared.

When you are preparing for your surgery, you want to make sure you have the answers to some key questions. This will enable you to be as emotionally prepared as possible, as well as having the practical things organized.

See *Chapter 18: Post-Op Recovery* for more information. It has great suggestions on making your recovery as easy as possible. You will want to read this before you have surgery.

Full Medical History

Before your surgery, you will most likely meet with your surgeon. If they haven't already done so, they will take a complete medical history. They will be asking about any health problems you have had, any medication you are currently taking or have taken in the past, as well as any known allergies. Make sure you tell your surgeon about any natural supplements you are taking as well, as these can impact anesthesia and clotting.

Here are some of the questions they should ask you:

- Do you have any **allergies**?

- Have you had a **bad reaction to** antibiotics, anesthetic drugs or any other medicine?

- Do you have **prolonged bleeding** or **excessive bruising** when injured?

- Do you have a **connective-tissue disorder** such as rheumatoid arthritis, scleroderma, lupus erythematosis, or any other arthritis-like disorder?

- Do you have any **long-term illnesses**?

- Have you had any **recent illnesses**?

- Have you previously had surgery for **breast cancer** or **radiotherapy** to the breast?

- Have you had any **surgeries** before?

- Have you had **psychological** or **psychiatric illnesses**?

Stop Taking Certain Medications & Natural Remedies

You may be asked to stop certain medications prior to your surgery that may interfere with your surgery and recovery. Most commonly, patients are advised to stop taking non-steroidal anti-inflammatory drugs (known as NASAIDs), aspirin, and any medications containing aspirin.

If you are using natural remedies, you may need to stop these as well. These include garlic, ginseng, ginkgo, and St. John's Wort.

Unless advised differently, you should be able to continue to take most medications as per normal.

Questions for Your Surgeon

In the process of choosing your surgeon, you will have undoubtedly asked them a lot of questions (such as those suggested in *Chapter 14: Questions to Ask Your Surgeon*).

Here are some questions you may like to get answered that specifically relate to your surgery:

- What **medication** will I be given or prescribed after surgery? Do I need to fill any prescriptions prior to surgery?

- What **dressings/bandages** will I use after surgery? If so, when will they be removed? Once I am home, how often do I need to change my dressings and what does that involve?

- What type of **stitches** will I have? Are the stitches removed? When will they be removed?

- When can I resume normal activity and **exercise**?

- When do I return for **follow-up care**? When do I need to book appointments?

- How soon can I **drive** after surgery?

- Do I need to bring my own **bra** to wear home or is one provided?

- What do I need to **buy** in terms of bandages, dressings, or creams?

- How soon after surgery can I **shower**?

- When can I have **sex** again?

Packing for Surgery

You won't need much while you're in hospital or your surgical center. Here's a quick guide of what to bring with you:

- Toiletries – toothbrush, toothpaste, moisturizer (you probably won't be up to washing your hair so you don't need shampoo and conditioner)

- Bathrobe (you probably won't need PJs as you will be

wearing a hospital gown)

- Cell/mobile phone

- Phone charger

- Headphones (in case you want to listen to music)

- Book or magazine (you probably won't be up to reading, but you never know)

- Clean underwear

- Compression bra

- Clothes to wear home (you won't be up to moving your arms above your head, so get a wrap dress/top, or something with zips or buttons)

- Thongs/flip flops/slippers for wearing to the bathroom

- Make-up (this is for when you leave the hospital – it might make you feel more human, but you may not be up to wearing make-up)

- Sanitary pads if you have your period

Menstruation & Surgery

Some women have their period at the time of their surgery. This is a double-whammy! You need to know that you are not able to use tampons during the actual surgery and will be required to use pads. Some surgeons will allow you to use a menstrual cup. Make sure you have a supply of menstrual pads.

Of course, if you have a regular menstruation cycle, you may want to consider having your surgery when you won't be menstruating.

CHAPTER 17

The Day of Your Surgery

Regardless of whether you've had surgery before, you will probably be a little anxious before your surgery. That's completely normal. You may also have some excitement mixed in with the nervousness, especially if you've been dreaming of a breast reduction for a long time.

Some people have never had surgery, broken a bone, or had stitches before. If this is you, please know that it is normal to feel fear in the face of the unknown. Knowing what to expect, at least intellectually, can help calm your fears somewhat. However, please discuss your anxiety with your surgeon as they can help allay your fears.

Here's an idea of what generally happens on the day of surgery:

Step 1: Change into hospital gown

Step 2: Meet with surgeon and have breasts marked up

Step 3: Have photographs taken of your breasts

Step 4: Have your IV line inserted

Step 5: Anesthesiologist visits to discuss anesthesia

Step 6: Go to operating theater and go to sleep

Step 7: Have surgery

Step 8: Wake up in recovery

Step 9: Transfer to your room (if day surgery, you will be discharged instead)

Step 10: Get discharged and go home

Please note the steps may vary according to the surgeon, where you are having your surgery, and even what country you are in. However, these steps give you a good idea of what to expect on the day.

Step 1: Gown Up

- When you arrive at the hospital or surgery center, you will be taken to a pre-op area. This could be a private room, a ward with curtains, or a waiting area. Depending on their policy, some places allow you to have your family with you in this area, some don't.

- You will be given a robe/gown and told to disrobe. You may be able to keep your underpants/panties on, so please check.

- You may be given a surgical cap to cover your hair. You may be asked to put it on as soon as you are in your gown, or you may put it on when you are about to be transported to the operating theater.

- You may also be given surgical slippers that you can either put on when you change into your gown or just before you are transported to the operating theater.

- Your bag and personal items may be put in a locker or straight into your room.

- After you have undressed, and you are in your hospital

gown, the surgeon will come and see you.

Step 2: Surgeon Visits and Marks Your Breasts

- The surgeon will use a texta or marker pen to do the surgical markings on your breast.

- You should only be asked to uncover the area being operated on, so you should retain your privacy.

- Depending on the establishment, you may have a nurse in the room with you. If for some reason you feel uncomfortable, you can request a nurse to be present.

- You may be seated or standing while the markings are being done.

Step 3: Photographs Are Taken

- The surgeon may take photographs of your breasts after the markings are done (sometimes they do this before). Most surgeons will also take pictures in your pre-surgery consultation so that they have the before photos.

Step 4: IV Inserted

- A nurse or the anesthesiologist will start your IV (intravenous line). Usually, a catheter is inserted into the back of your hand (normally the hand you do not write with). This can sting a little depending on the veins in your hand.

- An IV enables rapid absorption and precise control over the dosage of the substance administered. In your surgery, the IV will be used to deliver a saline solution, pain relief (such as morphine), and antibiotics if needed for some reason.

- With an IV, a small hollow needle is inserted into your vein. This needle has a very thin tube inside it. Once the

IV is in place, the needle is removed, leaving the tube inside your vein.

- The IV site will be taped to prevent this tube from falling or being jarred. (It can definitely hurt if it is knocked.)

- Once the IV tube is in, the tubing is connected to a bag that hangs from a hook on your bed or a stand with wheels on it.

- At this point, only a saline solution will be delivered via the IV. This is for hydration purposes and will not affect the way you feel.

Step 5: Anesthesiologist Visits

- Most likely this is the first time you have met your anesthesiologist. They will ask you some questions about your medical history such as whether you are pregnant (if you are, then this might not be the time for surgery!), past experiences with anesthesia, and whether you have any allergies. Even if you have answered these same questions with your surgeon, the anesthetist will ask them also.

- Your anesthesiologist will also ask if you have had anything to eat or drink in the last so many hours. You will be advised before coming to the hospital about the requirements for fasting (normally it is from midnight the evening before your surgery).

- It is key that you are totally honest with your anesthesiologist. If you don't tell them the truth, it could lead to serious consequences during surgery.

- Now is the time to ask any questions you have about the anesthesia. Breast reduction surgery is nearly always performed under general anesthetic.

- In an operating theater, the anesthesiologist is in charge of monitoring your vitals and making sure you are doing well during the surgery.

102

Step 6: Off to Theatre

- If you need to go to the bathroom, now is the time to do it!

- You will be transported to the operating theater. You may be asked to walk there, taken on a bed, or taken in a wheelchair.

- You will get onto or be transferred to an operating table. These are often quite narrow and are generally covered with a sheet.

- Normally, an operating theater is quite cold. You may feel a chill in the air. You may be given a heated blanket.

- Depending on the type of operating table, you may put your arms on rests which extend from the side of the table. You may also have your wrists secured to the rests with straps.

- The anesthesiologist or a nurse will attach a blood pressure cuff to your arm, and EKG leads (these are stick pads with little nubs on the ends that monitor your heart during surgery), a pulse oximeter (this is a plastic clip attached to your fingertip used to measure the amount of oxygen in your blood during surgery).

- The anesthesiologist, or a nurse, will put a mask over your face and ask you to breathe deeply.

- The anesthesiologist will inject anesthetic into your IV. This may burn or feel cold or tight at the site of your IV.

- Lights Out: this should be the last thing you remember until you wake up in the recovery room.

Step 7: The Surgery

You won't have any idea what is going on this phase. You will be knocked out. But here's what will happen:

- The surgeon will make incisions on the lines drawn earlier.

- Excess skin and glandular and fatty tissue will be removed.

- The areola may be resized.

- The nipple and areola will be positioned higher on the breast.

- Then the skin beneath the areola complex is brought together and closed together with dissolvable sutures to reshape the breast (some surgeons will use external sutures on the outside of the incisions as well).

- Before closing the breast completely, a surgical drain may be placed inside each breast to allow fluids to drain as they heal.

- Surgical tape or bandages will be applied to the incisions.

- You may be wrapped in a compression or elastic bandage (some surgeons just put your surgical bra or compression bra on you instead of a bandage).

Step 8: Wake Up in the Recovery Room

- A few hours later (often between two and five hours) you will wake up in the recovery room.

- You may feel nauseous. If you do, let your nurse know. You may be given some medication to reduce the nausea.

- Your surgeon will visit you in recovery to check how you are doing. They may tell you how the surgery went.

- Nurses will be keeping a good eye on you in recovery.

- Pain relief will be administered via your IV.

- Most people don't remember much about recovery as

they are quite out of it.

- How long you stay in recovery depends on how well you come out of the anesthesia, your blood pressure, heart rate, and blood oxygen levels as well as your surgery site. If there are any issues, you will stay in recovery for longer.

- No visitors are allowed in the recovery room.

Step 9: Off to Your Room

- When you are ready, you will be taken to your room. This may or may not be private. You can normally have visitors in your room.

- You should not be in any pain at this point. You will be getting pain medication via your IV.

- If you do feel pain, let your nurse know and she can adjust your pain medication.

- Some hospitals have self-administered pain relief, such as morphine. Your nurse will show you how to do it and how often you should be doing it.

- You will be weaned off the IV pain medication and onto pain relief pills.

- You may be thirsty and hungry by now and may be offered food and drink.

- Just drink and eat plain things, especially if you are still feeling queasy from the anesthesia.

- Your surgeon should visit you before you are discharged. They will examine your wound site and you can ask any questions about your surgery.

Step 10: Discharge Time

- If you have had drains in your wounds, they will be removed before you are discharged.

- If you are being discharged the day of your surgery, you will be asked to urinate before you leave.

- You will be asked to sign discharge papers.

- You will be given any prescriptions that you need.

- A follow-up appointment with the surgeon or another team member will be made. Normally you will have to come back in about three days to make sure that the wound is healing properly.

- Make sure you have the post-op care instructions.

- Have a family member or friend pick you up. You cannot drive.

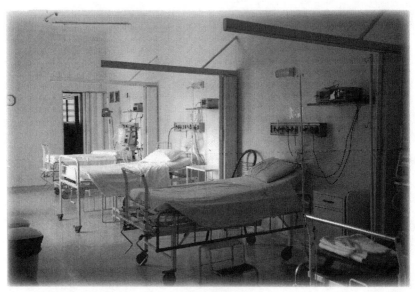

106

CHAPTER 18

Post-Op Recovery

You want to maximize your post-op recovery to ensure you have as little pain as possible, your surgical wounds are healing, and that you are feeling good about your surgery.

Here are some things you need to know about the recovery phase:

- Follow your surgeon's directions

- Contact your surgeon if you have any issues

- Make yourself a priority and rest up

- Set yourself up so that you can get a good night's sleep

- Work out a way to get out of bed that doesn't damage your wounds

- Organize your medical supplies so they are handy

- Be careful when you have your first shower after surgery

- Organize meals and snacks

- Stay hydrated and drink plenty of water

- Avoid alcohol

- Wear your compression bra

- Take a gentle laxative if constipated

- Avoid heavy lifting and excessive exercise

- Be prepared for post-op swelling and bruising

- Take arnica

- Use heat (and ice) packs with caution

- Understand that you first period post-surgery may be more painful

- Organize care of pets

Follow Your Surgeon's Directions

Your surgeon will provide specific instructions for post-operative care that may include:

- How to care for your breasts post-surgery

- Medications you need to take to aid healing and reduce infection

- Creams you need to apply to the wound and how to manage dressings

- Things to look out for as you are healing

- When to follow-up with your surgeon

Contact Your Surgeon

If you experience any of the following symptoms, contact your surgeon immediately:

- Temperature higher than 38ºC (100.4 Fahrenheit) or chills

- Nausea

- Vomiting

- Shortness of breath

- Diarrhea

- Heavy bleeding from the incisions

- Increasing pain or tenderness in either breast

- Leakage of blood or fluid beyond the first day after surgery

- Worsening and/or spreading redness around the incision sites

- Any other concerns or problems regarding your surgery, particularly if it appears to be worsening

Prioritize Yourself

You really need to take care of yourself at this time. Don't feel guilty that you aren't doing anything around the house or going to work. You need plenty of rest. Some people feel really out of it for about a week afterward. Remember that you have had major surgery and give yourself permission to lie around doing nothing (except maybe binge-watching Netflix).

If you are worried about your wound healing or anything else to do with your surgery, call the surgeon's office straight away. There are no stupid questions or concerns.

Rest Up

You're going to sleep a lot in the week or two after your surgery. Your body has been through a lot and it needs sleep to heal. Even if you're not asleep, you're going to be resting big time. Most people need two or three weeks to recover. You may be one of the lucky ones who feels great a week after surgery. But this is rare. Most likely you will feel like crap for at least two weeks. So be prepared to rest up.

Sleep Well

After your surgery, it is recommended that you sleep on your back. This will help wound healing. If you are a tummy sleeper, you may find this hard to adjust to. But it is necessary. There's no way you can sleep on your tummy after breast reduction surgery. Some people like to sleep in a recliner chair to recover in as they keep you slightly upright and you can't roll onto your side while you are in it. If you don't have one, you can rent them in some places.

You can put a pillow under each arm to create an armchair in your bed as well as a pillow under your knees (which will take the stress of your back). This is how I slept, and it worked very well. The pillows at your sides will support your arms while ensuring you don't roll over onto your side.

Some people rent hospital beds post-surgery. I don't think this is a necessity. The two pillows under the arms works fine for me. However, do see below on how to get out of bed.

If you're really struggling with lying on your back, just remember that you don't want to widen your incision. And if you want to prevent wrinkles, sleeping on your back is the best way to do it, so that's added motivation.

Get Out of Bed Safely

After surgery, you will be feeling weak. You will be limiting the use of your arms so that you don't strain your wounds, so getting out of bed can be a bit tricky when you only have minimal use of your arms.

When in bed, pull your knees towards your chest. Roll to the side and gently roll out of bed, careful not to roll onto your breast. Alternatively, pull your knees up and try to use a sit up type of motion and twist around to the side of the bed.

Having a nest of pillows on your bed can help you as they can prop you into a semi-upright position that can help you get out of bed.

The stronger your abdominal muscles, the easier you will find getting out of bed without using your arm muscles. If you do sit-ups in preparation for your surgery, this can help. Though, I don't imagine many will do this just for post-surgery recovery.

Have the Comfortable Clothes

After surgery, you don't want to be lifting your arms above your shoulders for a few weeks at least. Get yourself some tops that have buttons or zips, as well as some loose pants. Slip-on-shoes are also a good idea so that you don't have to bend down to put your shoes on. You aren't going to win any glamour awards, but at least you'll be comfortable.

Get Your Medical Supplies Organized

Get a bag or plastic tub that you can keep all your supplies in such as tape, ointment, and medication. Post-surgery, you won't be feeling the best, and you don't want to be looking for the things you need to care for your wounds and yourself.

Set a timer to take your medication. You may be drowsy and forget to take them at the right time.

Organize Your Home for Ease

There are several things you can do to make things around your house easier while you are recovering. Before you have your surgery, get anything you think you will need down from high shelves or cupboards. You don't want to be stretching to get a glass or a plate. Organize your TV remotes, books, and magazines, as well as anything else you think you might need so that you don't have to go searching for things.

111

Be Careful When You First Shower Post-Surgery

When you have your first shower after your surgery, be careful. You might get quite dizzy and could fall. Your center of gravity might be a bit off so take it easy. If someone can be in the bathroom while you shower, that would be great. If you do get dizzy, you can get them to assist you. If you have a shower over a bathtub, you may like to sit in the tub. You may also find that merely having a shower exhausts you. Plan to rest afterward.

Have Meals and Snacks on Hand

Hopefully, you have a good support network in place to help care for you while you are in the early days of recovery, at least for the first seven days. If you don't, make sure you have plenty of easy to prepare snacks and meals on hand. If you can make meals and freeze them before your surgery, that would be ideal. Also, have some fresh fruit and nuts in your kitchen.

Stay Hydrated - Drink Plenty of Water

Water is needed by every cell in your body. If you are dehydrated, your body will actually hold onto water, creating extra swelling. If you are retaining water due to dehydration, you may have more swelling and feel uncomfortable. So please make sure you are drinking enough water.

Soft drink/soda and coffee don't count; they dehydrate you. If you are not good at drinking water, try adding a squeeze and a slice of lemon or lime. This will make it taste more refreshing and help with healing.

Keep a bottle of water near your seat and bed. This way you can keep hydrated during the day without having to get up and down all the time. You may also like to have a thermos of warm tea beside your bed.

112

Take Laxatives If Needed

One of the side effects of anesthetic and pain medication can be constipation. Most people have a lot of trapped gas after surgery as well, so don't be surprised if you have some air pressure out your bum!

You may need to take a stool softener or gentle laxative to get things moving. Drinking plenty of water will also help.

Avoid Alcohol

Alcohol is one of those things you should avoid after surgery if you want to maximize your healing. Doctors recommend you abstain from alcohol for at least three weeks. You would be surprised to find out that many people have an allergic reaction to alcohol with excessive itching. This is probably due to the anesthesia and pain medications. Aside from the allergic reaction, alcohol can also impact healing.

Wear Your Compression Bra

Make sure you do wear your compression. It is a really important part of your healing process. It provides support for your breast while it is recovering.

Avoid Heavy Lifting & Strenuous Exercise

You don't want to do anything that is going to impact your wounds. Don't lift anything heavy, including children. And don't go running, lift weights or strenuous exercise. The most you should do is go for a gentle stroll around the block.

Be Prepared for Post-Operative Swelling & Bruising

Swelling is normal after surgery. Don't be surprised that you are so swollen around the surgery site. You will have bruises as well, especially if you've had liposuction. These bruises can be quite shocking, but it is your body healing. Excessive activity after surgery will also create more swelling.

Just remember, your body has been through major surgery and give yourself permission to heal.

The swelling around your breasts can last a long time after surgery. You may not be able to tell that you still have swelling, however, one sign is how your nipples appear in relation to your breasts overall. Swollen breasts often have nipples that appear to be pointing outward (like an eye that is lazy or crossed-eyed).

Another sign of swelling is that if your bra is leaving deep seam marks from wearing them, and they don't go away quickly once you take your bra off. Normal seam marks often disappear after a shower. Whereas with swelling, it can take over an hour for these seam marks to disappear.

See *Chapter 22: Nutrition for Recovery* for the Lemon Tea Recipe.

Take Arnica

Arnica has been shown to reduce pain, swelling, bruising and inflammation. It has natural anti-inflammatory properties. It increases circulation and stimulates white blood cell activity. This results in decreased healing time and reduced inflammation. Studies show that controlled doses of arnica can help reduce painful swelling.

You can get arnica in a cream or homeopathic tablet form. Post-surgery, the tablet is what you want as you won't be applying the cream to your fresh wounds. However, once the wounds are healed a little, you may be able to check with your surgeon to see if you can start applying arnica cream.

Many surgeons now provide arnica to their patients. My surgeon's practice recommended arnica post-surgery and even provided it to me. If your surgeon doesn't provide it through their practice, you can easily get it at any health food store as well as online.

Use Heat (and Ice) Packs with Caution

Many women love heats packs to help reduce pain. I love them myself. They are also very comforting. There is mixed advice about using heat packs post-surgery, so you may like to check with your surgeon.

Applying heat to your breasts may result in further swelling as the heat will dilate the soft tissues. Heat (and ice) can also affect blood flow to the breast, so you don't want to do any-thing to hinder the blood flow to the nipple.

Your breast area may be still numb post-surgery, so please use caution as apparently, lots of people burn themselves!

If you do use a heat pack, it is recommended that you only use them for a short period at a time and do not apply di-rectly to the skin (cover the heat pack with a tea-towel or something first). I mostly used heat packs on my lower back as lying around all day made my back sore.

Ice can be better than heat post-surgery because it can help decrease bruising, swelling and inflammation. Some surgeons recommend that patients apply ice packs over the top of their surgery bandages or bra at intervals of 15 minutes on and 15 minutes off. Just like heat packs, you want to be careful not to do damage (I imagine an ice burn isn't much fun).

Just check with your surgeon about what their preferences are.

Be Prepared for Increased Menstrual Symptoms

Many women are surprised to find that their first period after surgery is more painful than usual. This is because you are still healing from the trauma of surgery.

If you normally have breast tenderness before or during your period, you may find that your breasts are even more tender. If you often have stomach pain with your period, this may increase as well. If you normally don't have much tummy or breast pain around menstruation, you may have some the first period post-surgery. Drinking lemon tea can help relief.

Organize Care of Pets

Your loving dog or cat, or other pet, will undoubtedly want your affection and care. However, you want to make sure they don't jump all over you. Not only will it be painful, but it can also impact your recovery. Think about how you can still care for your pets while you are recovering. If you have a very large dog who loves to jump up on you, it might be wise to put them into a doggy hotel or have them stay outside if possible.

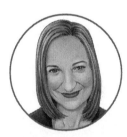

Ayesha: I was very blessed to stay with a close friend after my surgery. We had been bosom buddies for decades and had often discussed our large busts. My friend had had a reduction a few months earlier with the same surgeon.

When she had her surgery, I had visited her and supported her as best I could during her recovery. My friend knew exactly what to expect and helped me understand the breast reduction process. I felt well prepared and supported. I stayed with my friend for nearly two weeks. My husband at the time was in another town caring for our son and my daughter.

While I missed my children, I'm so glad I didn't have to care for them while recovering from surgery. I was sore. I was exhausted. And not up for much. If I wasn't in bed, my friend and I would lie on the couch binge-watching TV shows and movies. We got through two seasons of a Canadian TV show called Continuum.

CHAPTER 19

Post-Op Breasts

Seeing your new breasts for the first time will most likely be scary as hell and super exciting. I had longed to have a breast reduction for decades, so when it finally came to fruition, it was slightly surreal.

Will you fall in love with your smaller breasts?

Will you regret your reduction?

Or will you simply be in shock?

You need to know that the breasts you see right after surgery are not how your breast are going to look when they are fully healed. Remember, you've just had major surgery, and your breasts have had extensive trauma. It will take some time for them to recover.

Initially, your breasts will feel quite high on your chest and rather tight. As the swelling goes down, your breasts will most likely drop and round out.

The first thing many women wonder after their reduction is whether they have gone too small. After having such large breasts, you are used to seeing big boobs on your body. Big boobs were normal to you. It will take a while for your brain to adjust to seeing more petite breasts. Over time, the size and shape of your breast will normalize as will your perception of them.

We are not always the best judge of the actual size of our

breasts. You may feel like you're an A cup, but really you're a C cup. Alternatively, you may feel like you're a D cup, but really you're a C cup.

Remember, it's early days. Just breathe and be patient. And of course, talk to your surgeon and friends and family about how you feel if you're not happy with the result.

In my experience, many women are just so relieved to have smaller breasts, regardless of the size!

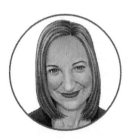

Ayesha: When I had my breast reduction, I felt like I was an A cup. It was so strange. They seemed too small. But to go from years of being an E, H and even an I cup (when breastfeeding) to a C cup made it seem like my breasts were an A cup!

Surgical Wounds

The wounds you have on your breasts will be dependent on the type of surgery you had. You will have stitches. You will have bruises. You will have swelling. And you will be as sore and tender.

Wound Breakdown or Scar Splitting

"Wound dehiscence, defined as significant wound breakdown which results in delayed healing (greater than 2 weeks), remains one of the most common complications after a breast reduction procedure. It constitutes a grievous complication for the patient and the surgeon."

http://www.medscape.com/viewarticle/822882_4

Wound breakdown is the most common problem faced by women after breast reduction surgery; as many as 50% of women experience some degree of wound breakdown. Most often, the wound will breakdown at the inverted T junction on the line that runs from your nipple vertically down to the bottom of your breast.

The wound or scar can begin to pull apart because of the tension on the wound edges. Infection can also cause your wound to breakdown. There are several factors that may contribute to a wound breakdown, such as poor diet, smoking, obesity, and long anesthetic times.

If you do have a wound breakdown, please contact your surgeon immediately so they can assess it. Treatment for wound breakdowns may vary by surgeon, but commonly includes the use of a topical antibiotic ointment (such as Neosporin) and non-adherent pads. Dressings need to be changed at least once a day after bathing. Alternatively, a Hydrofiber dressing such as Aquacel, can be used and this only needs to be changed every two or three days.

Wearing your post-surgery bra is important as this will help reduce the tension on the scar. When you have a wound breakdown, you need to be extra careful not to aggravate the wound or expose it to bacteria or germs.

In extreme circumstances, further surgical intervention may be required. This is not ideal, as it creates further tension needed to close the wound. There is a high chance of the wound breakdown occurring a second time in these situations.

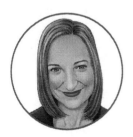

Ayesha: I wish I had known what a wound breakdown was before it happened to me. It was quite traumatic, especially as my surgeon was in another state, so I had to rely on my primary care doctor for advice about the wound healing process.

One breast had an open wound on it for months. It freaked me out; especially as I had no idea how long it was going to take to heal. I also couldn't have baths or go swimming. It eventually healed, but it took a few months. When it did heal, the scar on that breast was quite large where the wound breakdown had been.

Bottoming Out

Many women experience what is called *Bottoming Out*. This is where the lower part of the breast comes down with a loss of fullness in the top part of the breast and the nipple looks like it is pointing up. Often, bottoming out is caused by poor elasticity in the skin, the shape of the breast before surgery, or the surgeon's technique.

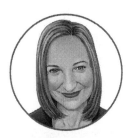

Ayesha: My breasts bottomed out. They are very flat in the upper pole, as my surgeon called it, before surgery. My surgeon suggested implants in the top part of my breast, but I declined.

Fat Necrosis

I didn't know about fat necrosis before I had my surgery. Necrosis is a scientific term defined by the Oxford Dictionary as *"the death of most or all of the cells in an organ or tissue due to disease, injury, or failure of blood supply."*

In breast reduction, this means that the fat cells die and clump together in the breast after surgery. These cells can form a lump in the breast that can be very small or as large as a grape or a golf ball. The lump is typically hard and dense, and can sometimes be confused with other lumps that are part of the healing process.

A fever is often associated with fat necrosis because a chemical is released during the death of the cells. The skin may also appear paler where the necrosis is occurring due to the decrease in blood supply.

Often the fat necrosis can break down on its own and be processed by the body. Good hydration and nutrition can aid the body in breaking down and releasing the necrosis, as can lymphatic support and lymphatic drainage massage.

If you do have signs of fat necrosis, speak to your surgeon. They should be able to assess whether it is fat necrosis or a lump that is just part of the healing process. If you do have fat necrosis, your surgeon may recommend that you gently massage the area to help break down the lump. This may be painful, so see how you go. In extreme cases, surgery might be required to remove the lump.

Even if you do have fat necrosis, this doesn't mean your breasts are ruined. It just may take some time for the lump to disappear.

Dog Ears

Normally a dog ear is the corner of a page turned down to mark your place. In plastic or cosmetic surgery, a dog ear refers to the puckering at the end of a scar. It is basically redundant tissue or skin. They are most commonly found at the end of skin-tightening incisions.

In breast reduction surgery, dog ears are normally found at the end of the breasts towards the armpits. It is like there is extra fat and skin at the end of your scar. The skin pokes out where it should be flat (thus the name dog ears).

Normally the use of liposuction on the outer part of the breasts is used to prevent dog ears. However, you can have liposuction and still develop dog ears. Many surgeons can predict who will likely get dog ears because of the amount of excess skin and the fatty deposits near the breast.

Sometimes dog ears may diminish during the healing process as the swelling reduces. Massage and steroid injections may also help.

Dog ears are typically corrected with minor scar revision. This is normally minor and done under local anesthetic. Most surgeons will not do a scar revision until the breasts have fully healed.

Some surgeons will do the corrective surgery as part of their whole package, while others may require additional payment to do the surgery.

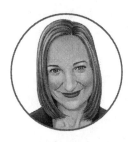

Ayesha: I have dog ears on both breasts. I had a lot of skin removed and my surgeon warned me that there was a high possibility of dog ears forming. I had the option to have them removed, but I decided not to. If you do develop dog ears, your surgeon should be able to correct them easily.

Melinda's Story

When I saw my breasts for the first time, I was in shock. They looked so small. Too small. What had I done? I was used to having big breasts and a nice cleavage. I had gone from an F cup down to a B cup.

While there were things I loved about having a breast reduction, it took me a long time to adjust emotionally to having smaller breasts. I felt like my breasts were too small for my body.

I discussed this with my surgeon. She said that there is often an adjustment period when a woman goes from large breasts to small ones. I definitely needed time to adjust.

It took me six months to feel comfortable with my new breasts. I wish I had gone a size larger, like a C cup. I do miss having cleavage. On the positive side, I can now wear push up bras and they do give a fairly good cleavage.

Even though I wish my boobs were a little better, I am more comfortable physically with smaller breasts.

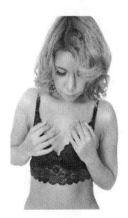

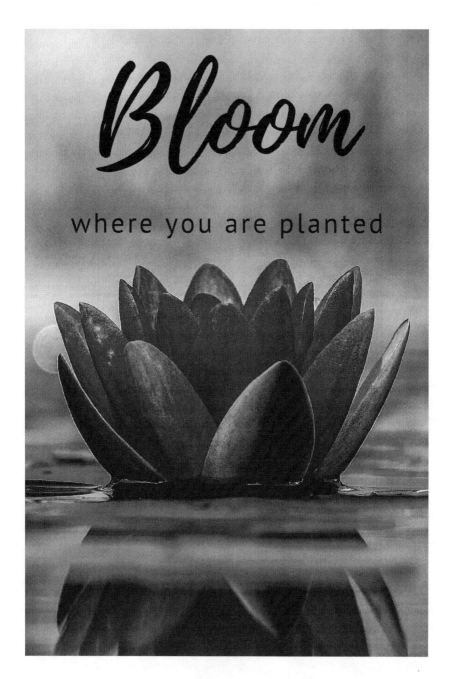

CHAPTER 20

Minimizing Scar Tissue

There are things you can do during your recovery, and over the 12 months after your surgery, that can help minimize scarring. Your surgeon should provide you with scar minimization protocols and post-op instructions.

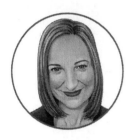

Ayesha: I have a lollipop scar that goes around the nipple and then down the front of the breast below the nipple as well as a long scar underneath each breast. Due to the amount of excess skin I had to have removed, my skin was more gathered and puckered by the sutures. These looked far worse in the beginning but do normalize six to twelve months' post-surgery. My scarring isn't bad at all now and I am quite happy with them. I do have dog ears on the outer part of each breast. I could have additional surgery to have these removed if I want.

Silicone Treatments

Silicone is used to help reduce scar on fresh wounds. It has been clinically tested to and proven to soften, flatten and smooth scars. Silicone also helps relieve itching and pain as the scar tissue heals.

American Academy of Dermatology and the International Advisory Panel on Scar Management recommend silicone therapy as the only non-surgical treatment for scar reduction.

The main role of silicone is to keep your wounds hydrated during the remodeling phase of the scar maturation. This allows the underlying cells to do their job more effectively.

There are three common ways for you to apply silicone: self-adhesive gel sheets, silicone tape, and silicone gel cream. Which one you use may be dependent on which one your surgeon recommends and what is most comfortable for you.

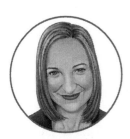

Ayesha: I used silicon tape after surgery and would change it every day or so. Make sure you dry it off gently with a towel after showering. I then moved onto the silicone cream once I no longer needed the tape. You can ask your surgeon what they recommend.

Post-Surgery Compression Bra

Before your surgery, you will be advised to purchase a couple of compression bras either through your surgeon, a bra shop, or an online store. These are the same types of bras used by women after having a mastectomy due to breast cancer.

While these bras are far from sexy and for some reason often come in beige, they serve a very serious purpose. The compression bra helps decrease swelling and post-operative pain. It also helps remodel soft tissue and helps to contour the breast.

The bra is worn day and night following surgery. Your surgeon will advise you how long you need to wear the bra. Some surgeons advise two to three weeks, while my surgeon recommended six weeks.

Most people are able to wear the bra comfortably during this time – as long as you have the right size. If it is cutting off circulation or is very uncomfortable, make sure you've got the right size.

Once you finish wearing the compression bra, you can move onto a sports bra for an additional six weeks. You can then start wearing a normal bra after this, but do not wear an underwire until you are fully healed. Many surgeons recommend not wearing an underwire bra for at least six months. And trust me, with smaller breasts; you won't mind not having an underwire bra. Before my breast reduction, I could not wear a bra that didn't have underwire.

Good Nutrition

You need to take care of yourself before and after surgery to ensure that your body has the best possible nutrients to help with the healing process. Fresh fruits and vegetables are your best friends in your recovery. If you don't have someone to cook for you during recovery, you may like to make up batches of soup and other healthy meals in advance. You may also need to increase your intake of essential vitamins and minerals.

See *Chapter 22: Nutrition for Recovery* for more information on maximizing your nutrition.

Post-Op Scar Massage

Massage can really help your healing. You need to check with your surgeon to see when you can begin massage and apply cream to your incisions.

Massage is recommended post-surgery because it:

- Promotes collagen remodeling by applying pressure to the scars

- Brings oxygen to the area that helps healing

- Helps decrease itching

- Provides moisture and pliability to the area

Scar Massage Technique

Once you have the ok from your surgeon, here is how to massage your scars:

- Apply a cream or lotion to the scar areas (I love coconut oil as it is antibacterial and very healing for the skin, but any unperfumed/unscented cream will work)

- Massage the cream or oil into the skin

- Apply enough pressure with the pads of your fingers to make the scar area turn white

- Massage in three different ways:

- *Circular* motions (you can do clockwise or counter-clockwise or both)

- *Vertical* motions (up and down)

- Horizontal motions (side to side)

Repeat two to three times per day. You may like to do it after you have your morning shower and before you go to bed, as well as one other time a day.

Alternatively, you may like to do your massage in the shower. You can use some soap or oil. The key is to do the massage. Find a way for you to do it every day; products don't matter as much as the massage itself.

Preventing and/or Treating Keloid Scarring

Treatments for keloid scar tissue can include surgery to remove the scar (though how effective this would be on the breast area is questionable), steroid injections, and the use of silicone sheets to flatten the scar. Small scars can sometimes be treated with cryotherapy (freezing the scar with liquid nitrogen). The best way to prevent keloid formation is to use pressure treatment or gel pads with silicone.

Fraxel Laser Scar Minimization Treatments

Fraxel Laser treatments are used to help reduce scars. In the US, the FDA has approved Fraxel Lasers, and there may be other laser treatments available. Always make sure you go to a professional. While laser treatment can aid with scar reduction, some people report that there was no change in their scarring after treatment.

I know a woman who had quite bad keloid scarring after her reduction. She was very committed to minimizing her scarring, so she did silicone treatments, massage, and ate very well. She then opted to have laser treatment. Unfortunately, the laser treatment made her scarring worse.

So, then the question becomes, would you prefer to have large breasts or keloid scars? When I asked this of the woman with severe keloid scarring, her answer was a resounding yes to having the scars. So even though she's got bad scarring, she's still happier having smaller breasts.

> *"Before I had the surgery, men were talking to my chest the entire time, but I couldn't blame them. When I walked into a room, my breasts were always several steps ahead of me."*
> *Mimi Rogers*
> *Actress*

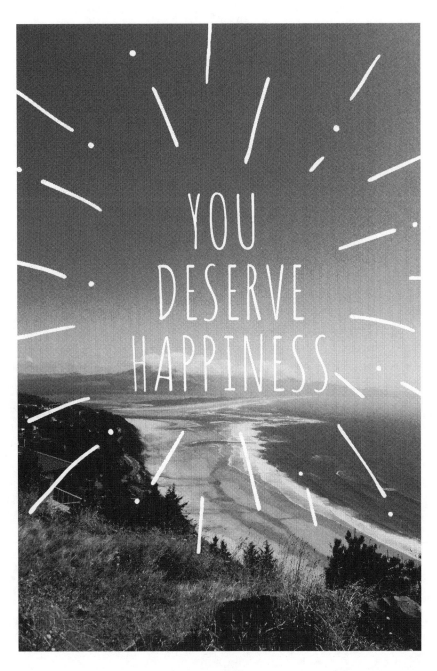

CHAPTER 21

Itching & Burning

You should know that your scars may start to itch and possibly burn within the first two weeks or so. And sometimes, the itching and burning can return sporadically weeks or months later.

This itching and burning is very common. It doesn't necessarily mean anything is wrong. So, don't freak out if your boobs start driving you nuts!

Most people say that itching is a sign of healing and that burning is a result of nerve generation. However, this is not the complete picture. Itching can be a sign from your body that you need better nutrition to help you heal. (See *Chapter 22: Nutrition for Recovery* for more information on maximizing your nutrition.)

It may also mean that you are having a reaction to something such as medication, adhesive tape, bandages or surgical glue. Or it could be an adverse reaction to alcohol in any form (even cough medicine). Alcohol is not your friend during the first few weeks after surgery because of all the medication in your system.

If alcohol is a trigger, please wait a few more weeks before consuming anymore. You shouldn't really be drinking in the first four to six weeks post-surgery if you want to optimize your recovery. Alcohol impacts healing by reducing your nutritional intake and it also thins your blood. Many surgeons recommend not drinking for four months after surgery.

You might need to put your detective hat on to see if something is exacerbating the itching and whether there are any other symptoms (such as a rash or flushing of the skin). Look at whether it gets worse after taking a specific medication or using adhesive tape on your scars. Or it might even be your sutures.

The key is to notice what is going on with your body, identify anything that makes the itching worse, and to discuss it with your surgeon. Sometimes, itching is a sign of a severe allergic reaction and needs to be treated immediately. If you find yourself suddenly extremely itchy, call you surgeon or go to the emergency room.

If in doubt, call your doctor! I'd rather be safe than sorry.

Here are some tips for managing your itching so that you don't go insane:

- Apply cool or warm washcloths or face washes to your itching skin. (Please get permission from your surgeon before applying heat to your incisions.)

- Use an anti-itch cream approved by your surgeon.

- Set a hairdryer on cool and move it quickly over the itching area.

- Wear a different bra or put a soft cotton t-shirt under your bra.

- If you have permission to go bra-free, don't wear one and just have your breast uncovered for a while.

- Put slight pressure on the itchy area with your fingers. Don't rub though.

Sophie's Story

My breast reduction surgery went well and I recovered easily. I was taking good care of myself and my scars. I had laser treatment to reduce the scars, and I used a topical silicon cream daily.

A couple of months after my surgery, my scars started to change and grow thicker. They also started to itch a lot. I contacted my surgeon and had an appointment. I had developed keloid scars.

Today, two years down the track, my scars are very raised, red, and often itchy. When I told a friend recently about my scars, she was horrified, but I told her that I would still prefer to have keloid scars than to have my large breasts.

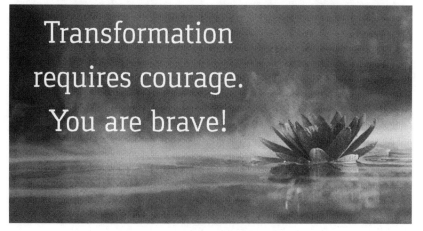

Transformation
requires courage.
You are brave!

133

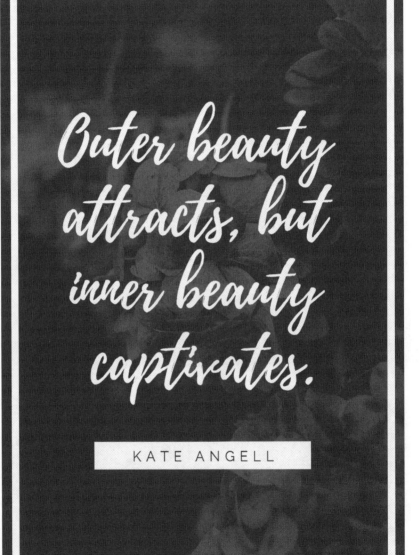

Outer beauty attracts, but inner beauty captivates.

KATE ANGELL

CHAPTER 22

Nutrition for Recovery

Good nutrition will really help your recovery. And poor eating and drinking will slow your healing down.

Here are general recommendations for maximizing your healing through nutrition:

- Eat plenty of fresh fruits and vegetables

- Drink plenty of water (with a slice/squeeze of fresh lemon or lime)

- Get enough protein

- Get enough vitamins and minerals (Vitamin C, Vitamin A, Zinc, and Iron)

- Avoid foods that cause an adverse reaction

To maximize healing, I suggest you avoid:

- Processed foods as much as possible

- Soda/soft drink

- Too much sugar (sugar will reduce your immune function for hours after you eat)

- Alcohol

Get Plenty of Protein

Protein is essential for healing post-surgery as it will help rebuild damaged skin, collagen and blood vessels. Lack of protein will slow healing down. So, if you want your surgical wounds to heal as quickly as possible, consume healthy protein such as meat, poultry, fish, beans, and eggs.

Vitamin C

Vitamin C is also integral to healing. Wounds heal in a step-by-step process that begins with collagen. As collagen is formed, new skin then grows in from the edges of the cut, using collagen for support until it meets in the middle. While collagen is made from protein, its production depends on the presence of Vitamin C. Good sources of Vitamin C include citrus fruit and juices as well as strawberries, tomatoes, capsicum/peppers, broccoli, spinach, cabbage, brussels sprouts as well as baked potatoes (not fries/chips). You may also like to take a daily dose of Vitamin C supplement.

Vitamin A

Like Vitamin C, Vitamin A is important to the healing process. Vitamin A is a powerful antioxidant that fights inflammation and supports skin and cell growth. It boosts the initial inflammatory response to the trauma of surgery. This is important at the beginning of wound healing to prevent infection. The inflammatory response in your body will get rid of any harmful irritants and bacteria. Vitamin A also helps stimulate collagen synthesis.

Vitamin A is found in eggs, whole milk, livers (if you're up to eating them) yellow and orange vegetables (such as carrots, squash, pumpkin), and dark green leafy vegetables like spinach.

Please note that high doses of Vitamin A can be dangerous and do more harm than good. Getting Vitamin A from food sources is your best option. However, if you take a Vitamin A supplement, please speak to your healthcare professional to make sure you are getting the right dose.

Zinc & Iron

Zinc is essential to wound healing because your body can't produce protein and collagen without zinc. Iron delivers oxygen to the wound site. One of the most common causes of infection after surgery is a lack of oxygen. So, you want to make sure your iron levels are good. Protein-rich foods are a good source of both zinc and iron. Whole grains and fortified cereals and bread also have zinc and iron.

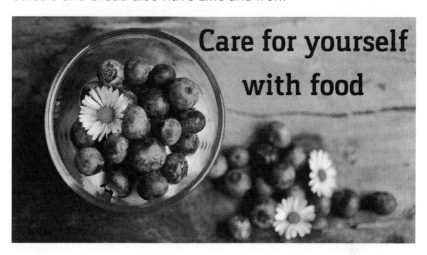

Care for yourself with food

Avoid Foods You Know Cause a Bad Reaction

If you have any food intolerances, try to avoid those foods while healing. An inflammatory response to food will slow your healing down. I personally have issues with gluten and dairy.

Drink Lemon Tea

You may like to try Annette's Lemon Tea (from Breast-HealthOnline.org) to help with your swelling and general recovery.

Drink one or two cups of this tea before bed at night, and you will see a marked improvement in your swelling in the morning. It is especially helpful to tender breasts during your first post-op menstruation.

Ingredients

To make lemon tea, you will need:

- One whole fresh lemon (not bottled or in the lemon shaped containers, but Minute Maid frozen is great)

- One cup of hot/boiling water

- Sugar/honey/molasses to taste (no artificial sweeteners)

Directions

- Using firm pressure, roll the lemon on a table or counter

- Cut the lemon in half, squeeze the all the juice

- Mix juice and one cup of hot water

- Sweeten to taste

1-2 cups a day are sufficient. It can be made cold (lemon-ade) if you prefer.

Despite being acidic, lemon juice has an alkalizing effect on your body once it has been consumed.

Many people worry about the acidity of drinking lemon juice. So here are Annette's recommendations for avoiding acidity issues:

- Don't brush your teeth right after drinking this (it softens the enamel)

- Drink through a straw, so you avoid the lemon touching

your teeth

- Rinse your mouth with clean water

- Avoid cleaning your teeth for a few hours

Katie's Story

Breast reduction surgery was the best decision I ever made (aside from choosing to marry my lovely husband)! I don't hurt every day. My back pain is completely gone. I'm just so much more comfortable in my body. And people aren't gawking at my breasts all the time. It is so much fun to shop for pretty bras and clothes that actually fit.

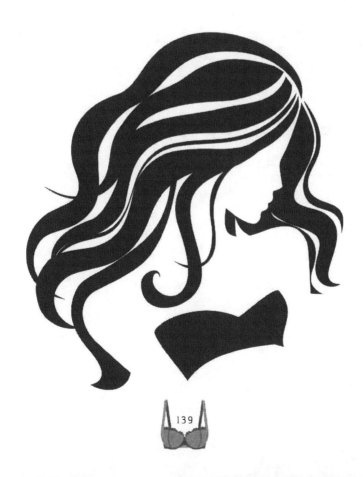

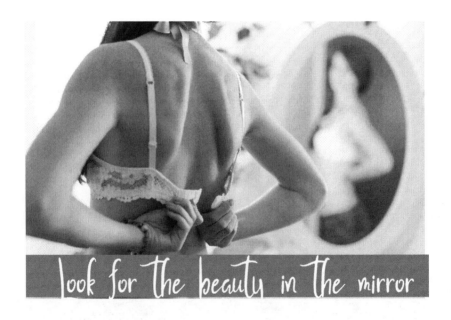

look for the beauty in the mirror

CHAPTER 23

Post-Op Blues

Post-op blues are common for any surgery patients. In most cases, the depressed mood is temporary and resolves itself within a couple of weeks. If your depression lasts longer than two weeks, please contact your surgeon or healthcare provider.

Breast reduction is major surgery of a large and sensitive area. It can take a lot longer to recover than you imagined. You have to make sure you take time to rest and heal. Many women are surprised to go through a blue period at some stage after surgery. It is often a shock because you've finally got what you wanted for so long!

While you may be excited about the changes in your breasts, you may also have some mixed feelings. You may be in pain. Your breasts may not look like you imagined (remember the swelling takes a long time to go down). You may also have anxiety about how others will perceive you, especially your partner if you have one. This is all normal.

There is also a delay in celebrating and enjoying your new boobs because the recovery takes so long. Just be patient. You've probably had large breasts for a long time and before you know it, the recovery period will be over.

Manage Your Post-Op Blues

Not everyone feels blue after their surgery, but if you do:

- **Don't Beat Yourself Up**

It's normal to feel a bit blue after so much change and pain.

- **Cry & Share Your Feelings**
  Give yourself permission to cry and talk about it with a family member or friend who will listen and support you. Expressing your feelings generally helps you feel better.

- **Journal Your Feelings**
  You may like to keep a breast reduction journal. You are going through a major life change. Write down your feelings and thoughts.

- **Stay Hydrated**
  Make sure you are drinking plenty of water. You have had a lot of medication in your system, and this can affect your mood. Water will help flush out the medication and toxins from your body.

- **Eat Well**
  As mentioned previously, good nutrition will help you heal. And it will also help your mood.

- **Rest & Relax**
  Many women find it hard to rest and relax. You've had major surgery and your body needs time to heal. Get someone to give you a foot massage. Read an inspiring book. Watch the clouds roll by.

- **Laugh**
  Laughter is the best medicine for the blues. Many people don't realize that they have the power to change their mood through laughing. If you're feeling blue, go to YouTube and watch funny cat videos. Or watch a rom-com on Netflix and laugh. When you laugh, you change your brain chemistry, and you start to feel better.

- **Allow Yourself to Receive Help & Support**
  As women, we are used to taking care of others and doing a lot in our lives. And if you're a mother, you are used to managing the household and taking care of everyone. Give yourself permission to let others help and support

you. You may even pay someone to come and clean your house if you need.

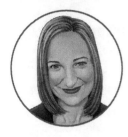

Ayesha: Before I had breast reduction surgery, I would look enviously at the smaller sized bras in the shops. They were much prettier that the massive bras I needed.

I was so excited to know that I could finally have gorgeous lingerie instead of beige grandmotherly bras. Wait to go out and buy cute new bras until you've had time to heal. I didn't wait, and now I have a cupboard full of bras that don't fit properly.

I know that many people keep their breast reduction a secret. I wrote a blog post and shared it on Facebook, so it wasn't a secret. Whether you tell other people or not, is totally up to you. It's your body, your choice. Though if it is a secret, be prepared for people to notice or comment, especially if there is a big change in bust size.

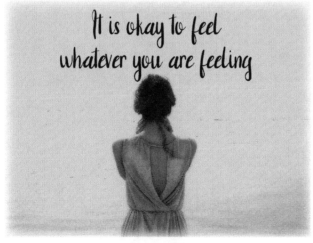

It is okay to feel
whatever you are feeling

143

The Story of Ariel Winter
Star of Modern Family

Ariel Winter is the gorgeous actress who stars in the US sit-com Modern Family. She grew up on TV and was quite young when she started. As she got older, her breasts got bigger. At age 15, she was wearing an F cup. Her breasts caused a lot of back pain. The females in Ariel's family have a history of large breasts.

Ariel decided to have surgery after she went swimwear shopping with her cousin. She couldn't find anything to fit her and was frustrated and sad that she couldn't wear normal bathers.

Even though breast reduction isn't normally recommended for girls as young as 17, Ariel was so uncomfortable; she knew she had to have surgery. In June of 2015, Ariel had breast reduction, going from a 32F to a 34D.

She reported noticing a difference straight away. She told glamour magazine that she felt like a new person and could now dress in clothes appropriate to her age.

Ariel attracted a lot of attention when she first hit the red carpet after her breast reduction. She handled it with poise well beyond her years.

CHAPTER 24

Caring for Small Children

Motherhood is full-on at the best of times. If you're having breast reduction surgery and you have young children, keep reading because it's a lot harder to get the rest you need, and you will need it!

My son was only three, and my daughter eight, when I had my surgery; I chose to recuperate away from home for ten days. This was a complete luxury, one that I truly appreciated. I knew I couldn't care for my children properly, and if I were at home, I would want to do stuff around the house, and my son would want to jump on me for cuddle time. I must say, it was a good choice, but by day eight, I was desperate to have some cuddle time with my beautiful munchkins. And I think my husband was ready for me to return too.

Most of the women I know haven't had the choice to recuperate away from their children. In fact, many still end up caring for their children full-time. You need to prioritize rest, so there are several things you can do to make your recovery easier:

- Schedule your surgery at a time when you can get the most help

- Limit heavy lifting

- Get outside care or support if possible

- Ask your children to help out more

- Avoid lifting your child in and out of bed/cot

- Make meal times easy by getting take-out, packaged food, or preparing and freezing meals in advance

- Encourage children to dress themselves

- Change nappies/diapers on the floor or couch

- Get help with bath time or let your kids have a shower

- And think before you act – ask: "Will this be good for my recovery?"

- Give yourself a break and be compassionate to yourself

Top Tips for Mothers

Thank you to BreastHealthOnline.org for many of these great tips!

Schedule Your Surgery Wisely

- Schedule your surgery when you can get the most support from your partner, best friend, mother, and/or sibling. Also, if you have school-aged children, it would be preferential that your recovery be during the school year.

- If you have a partner/spouse/hubby, see if they take some time off work to help with the kids and the house. Ideally, two weeks would be great. But at least one week is needed.

- If you're a single parent, see if your kids can stay with grandparents for a few days or if you have a mother/sister/best friend who could stay and take care of you, that would be great.

Limit Lifting

You should also be aware of the following:

146

- The longer you wait to do lifting, the better.

- Check with your surgeon to see how long you need to wait before lifting your child or anything heavy. Most surgeons recommend at least six weeks.

- When you have "permission" from your surgeon to lift, be very careful when you lift and try to limit heavy lifting for a while. And of course, remember to bend your knees.

- You can injure yourself, opening your wounds or tearing something, if you lift too soon. Kids can weigh a ton, so take it easy.

Don't Try to Be a Super Mother

- Don't try to be a super mother! If your house is messier than normal and your kids eat less than ideal for a couple of weeks, give yourself a break. Your rest and recovery are your priorities right now.

- Leave the laundry and bath times for your partner.

- Get your kids to help more around the house.

- Before long you will be back to your normal self, and the house will be just the way you like it.

Outside Care

- If you have very young children, you may consider day care while you are recovering. This will cut down the number of hours you need to be responsible for the care of your children and allow you to get some much-needed rest.

- If day care is not available or an option, think about hiring someone locally to babysit for you.

- You may also like to consider getting some home help, such as a cleaner - or in the US, some insurance companies will pay for a home health aide. A home health aide is not a nurse. Their job is to do light housework, prepare and clean up after meals, grocery shop, and do laundry for you. Which sounds pretty good to me!

- If you are a member of a local church, you could ask some of the congregation to help out.

- Ask friends for casseroles and meals! People love to help and will be glad you asked, most of the time.

Ask Your Children to Help Out

- Children often love to help with jobs around the house. They are great at fetching things for you and lifting light things. My son helps me hang out the washing on a clothes horse as well as sorting the clothes into piles when they are dry.

- You can make a game of it!

Make Meals Easy

- Don't feel guilty or ashamed if you let your children's nutrition slide for a couple of weeks. It won't kill them. And honestly, you will not be up to slaving over a hot stove – trust me!

- If you don't have someone cooking for you each day, make sure you prepare plenty of meals in advance and pop them in the freezer. This will make it easy to simply reheat the meals and serve. You can either make up servings for just you (as your nutrition is really important during recovery) or for the whole family.

- Packaged foods might be your savior during this time. Don't worry; it's just for a short time. Frozen meals or microwavable meals can feed hungry mouths while not sapping all your energy.

- We like to have breakfast dinners. We have toast and

eggs and maybe hash browns and bacon for the meat eaters. These are fun, delicious and quick.

- Take away (or take out) meals are another good option if you have the budget for them. And you can quickly reheat leftovers later. Of course, try and choose healthier takeaway meals.

- If your child eats in a highchair normally, why not put a booster seat on the floor to feed them. This means you don't have to lift them into a highchair.

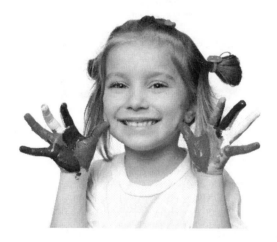

Avoid Lifting at Nap/Bed Times

- To help your child into their bed or cot, use a small stool or ladder. You do not want to be lifting them! And your child might really like it.

- If your child is almost ready to transition from a cot to a toddler bed, you could do it before your surgery. Make it a celebration!

- Let your child nap on the floor on a small blanket. You can both have a rest!

Encourage Your Children to Dress Themselves

- This is the perfect time for your little ones to start dressing themselves.

- If your child still needs your help, sit on the couch and have them stand or kneel in front of you. You want to limit lifting and putting your arms above your shoulders.

- Prepare outfits (tops, pants, undies, etc.) in advance and put them where your child can reach them. Each morning they can help themselves to a new outfit.

- BreastHealthOnline.org has a cool idea – put a rubber band around each outfit to keep them together.

Changing Nappies/Diapers without Lifting

(For the US people, we call diapers "nappies" here in Australia.)

- The aim is to not lift your child. Your two best options are the couch or the floor. If they can climb, get them to get on the couch. If they can't, just change them on the floor. You can use a towel to put under their bums!

- Roll your child onto the nappy, rather than grabbing their legs and feet and lifting them. Remember, no lifting, mama!

Manage Bath Time

- Firstly, your children probably don't need a bath every day. So, don't fret if they miss a day or two.

- Secondly, if you have a partner or someone else helping you, let them manage bath time and put your feet up.

- DO NOT, I repeat, DO NOT, lift your kids in and out of the bathtub. You can do real damage, especially in the first ten days or so.

- If you don't have any other options for bath time, let your children have a big boy or big girl shower!

- My son wasn't into showers initially, but now he loves them. This is what I did, I got him his own shower cap and toys to play with. If your child doesn't like water in the eyes, why not give them some goggles to wear in the shower.

Think Before you Act

Please take care of yourself. Ask yourself if this action will be detrimental to your healing. If so, find another way. Use your creativity and have fun with your kids. Turn limitations into a game. Before you know, you will be back to your normal self, and your children won't be damaged by the few weeks you took off from being a superhero mother!

Be Compassionate to Yourself

You are giving yourself such a gift by reducing your bust size. Don't screw it up over-doing things. Life doesn't have to be neat and tidy while you're recovering. You won't be up to reading ten books a night or going to the park and pushing your child on the swing for hours. And that's ok. Give your-self permission to put yourself first for this short period. If you've waited years for surgery and possibly put it on hold until you finished breastfeeding, like I did, this is your time! You deserve it!

Give yourself permission to take care of yourself and allow others to support you

Rachel's Story

I didn't have children until quite late in life. I'd dated a lot of good men but didn't find the one I wanted to settle down with until I was 35. Brian and I got married and had children quite quickly. In the space of five years, I'd gone from being a single, career-focused woman, to being a stay-at-home mum with two children under the age of three. My life was busy and chaotic, but I was happy.

The only thing really affecting my happiness was my breasts. I'd always had large breasts, but with pregnancy weight gain and two years of breastfeeding, my breasts were in bad shape. After I stopped breastfeeding, my breasts, which had grown considerably larger, were very droopy. I had a lot of skin on the top half of the breast and it was very flat. Without a bra on, my breasts nearly went down to my belly button. I loved that my breasts had fed and nurtured my children, but now when I looked at them, they seemed to belong to the body of an old woman.

One day, I was having coffee with a friend and was mourning the loss of my youthful breasts. My friend confided that she knew exactly what I was talking about and confessed that she'd had a breast reduction a couple of years earlier. I had no idea she'd had a reduction. I asked her question after question. I'd not thought of having a breast reduction (and a lift), but the idea got stuck in my head and I couldn't let the idea go.

My husband and I spoke about it. He loves me just the way I am and didn't mind my sagging boobs. But he wanted me to have a breast reduction if it was what I wanted. I found a surgeon, and before I knew it, I was booked in for surgery.

152

The surgery went well, and I was home before I knew it. Alas, I didn't really consider the impact of surgery on my ability to look after two young children. I couldn't change nappies or do bath times.

My husband ended up taking an unscheduled week off work to help as well as enlisting his mother to help out. I was so tired; I could barely do anything for the first two weeks after surgery. If I had my time over, I would plan it better. I think my recovery would have been easier if I had. That said, I'm so happy with my breasts. They are so much smaller, but not too small, and they remind me of the breasts I had when I was in my late teens.

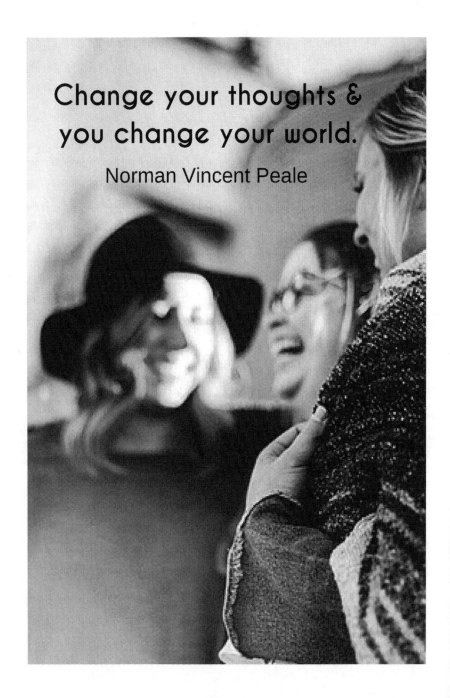

Change your thoughts &
you change your world.

Norman Vincent Peale

CHAPTER 25

Weight Changes & Your Breast Size Post-Surgery

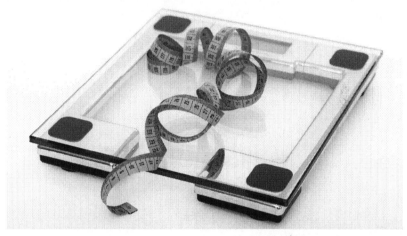

One of the most asked questions I've encountered is:

"What happens if I gain weight after my breast reduction surgery? Will my breast become huge again?"

Similarly, some women worry about what will happen to their breasts if they lose weight.

Despite having a breast reduction, your breasts can still be weight sensitive in either direction.

Breast reduction removes glandular breast tissue and fatty tissue. There is always some fatty tissue left in the breast, and this can grow as your body stores fat in the areas it is accustomed to, like the breast. If you gain weight, your breasts may increase in size. Likewise, if you lose weight, your breasts may get smaller and may create sagging skin.

155

How much your breasts will increase as a result of weight gain is dependent on the amount of fat tissue in the breast (and the older you are, the more fatty tissue there will be).

Most people do not notice any difference in breast size with small weight gains of less than 35 pounds.

One woman I know had a breast reduction in her early 20s, and then gained weight over the years. When she lost weight, she had a lot of excess skin. She had a second breast surgery.

If you get pregnant in the future, your breasts may also grow larger. Most women, whether they have had a breast reduction or not, will have breast growth during pregnancy, as their bodies are preparing for breastfeeding. Sometimes, breasts return to their pre-surgery size. This can be quite distressing for many women. However, most women's breasts return to their new size once they start breastfeeding.

If you are planning to lose weight, and feel confident that you will, you may consider waiting until after you lose weight to have your surgery.

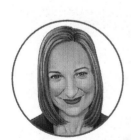

Ayesha: I have struggled with my weight for 20 years. When I had my surgery, I was at my ideal weight, and it was the perfect time for me to get my breast reduction so that I could get rid of as much skin as possible as well as breast tissue.

Not long after my surgery, my weight went up due to hormonal issues. I didn't really get to enjoy my new breasts at my ideal weight or the beautiful clothes I was looking forward to wearing.

I remember crying in my car after an appointment with my endocrinologist who'd just told me that there wasn't much I could do about my weight.

He prescribed weight loss drugs - like speed - but they didn't do anything for me. I gained more than 20 kilos (about 50 pounds) in a very short period. It was quite depressing and stressful. At the time of writing this book, I am at my heaviest. My breasts have gone up two bra sizes.

The one positive is that I didn't look as fat as I normally would have at this weight because my boobs are not massive. In the past, when I gained weight, my breasts would be the first place fat would go! The scars on the bottom of my breasts have moved up from the fold of my skin a little, and I have extra flab where the liposuction was done on the side of my breasts under my arms.

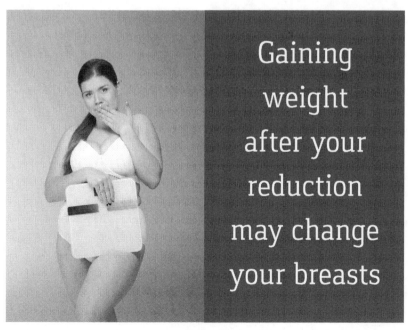

Gaining weight after your reduction may change your breasts

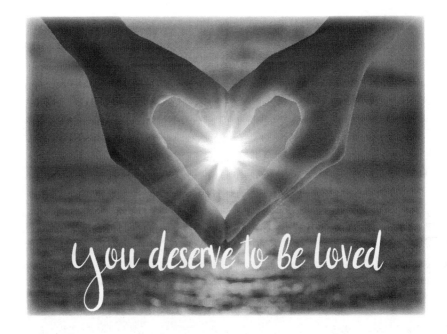

you deserve to be loved

CHAPTER 26

Talking to Your Partner

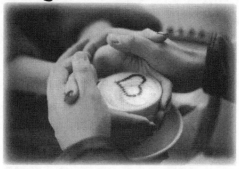

If you are in a relationship, talking to your partner about your desire to have a breast reduction is vital. They may be incredibly supportive straight away, or they may take a while to warm up to the idea.

Let them know why you need a breast reduction and what having one will provide you (such as feeling sexier, feeling more comfortable in your body, and having less physical symptoms).

Then ask them if they are willing to help support you on this journey as it would mean so much to you to have them by your side. Help them understand what you are going through and how they can best support you.

If you need your man's help, ask him for it outright. Don't rely on hints to get what you want. And appreciate him when he does help and support you. The more you appreciate him, the more he will be willing to help!

If you feel comfortable, share the following letter with the man in our life.

Dear Loving Partner

You have an amazing woman in your life. She's beautiful inside and out (even if she doesn't know it or feel it), and she's about to do something really important and life changing.

Perhaps she's been dreaming about breast reduction surgery for years. She may have even put it off to breastfeed your children. Maybe you've heard her complain of back and neck pain. Or perhaps lament the fact that she can't find a bra, top, or dress that fits her properly.

Breast reduction surgery is life changing. But it can also be challenging for many women. She may be worried that you won't view her the same way. Perhaps you like her big bust more than she does. Maybe you're worried she will change once she has surgery.

It's normal for both of you to be a little anxious or afraid. This is a big change, for both of you. Feel whatever you're feeling and be as honest as you can with your beautiful woman about what is coming up for you.

You have an important role in providing support to your woman through the breast reduction process. She needs you to be her hero during this journey. She may want you to go to the surgeon's office with you. She may want your help choosing a surgeon. And she will definitely need you to hold her hand as she goes into the hospital or day surgery center.

Your job is to provide her with support. She needs you. And she will love you even more than she already does for the kindness and support you show her.

She shouldn't be driving for a few weeks. And she can't do any lifting for at least six weeks. She may be in pain. She might be more emotional than normal due to the pain, the change in her body, and the pain relief medication. For the first week or two, she may be very tired and out of it. She will need a lot of rest.

160

There are plenty of things you can do to help her, and you may not need this list, but I will share it with you anyway:

- *Let her discuss any fears she may have (no matter how much she wants a smaller bust, she may still be afraid of the process and the results)*

- *Pick her up from her surgery, take her home, and help her get settled*

- *If you have young children at home, perhaps ship them off for the first night home to grandparents or friends*

- *Feel free to buy her flowers or chocolates*

- *Help around the house with the cleaning, dishes, laundry, and grocery shopping*

- *Do bedtimes and bath times with the kids*

- *Cook her meals, make her a cup of tea*

- *Massage her feet*

- *Tell her you love her and how beautiful she is*

I am sure there are plenty more things you can think of that will support your woman during this delicate time of healing.

Thank you for taking such great care of the woman you love.

Regards

Ayesha Hilton

Final Words

Breasts play such an important role in a woman's life. If you have been struggling with the pain and discomfort of large breasts for a long time, breast reduction surgery may be the very answer your prayers.

Surgery doesn't come without risks, and there are no guarantees that you will get the breasts you want. However, in talking to so many women about their breast reduction experiences, I have yet to find one who regretted having the surgery.

Many women who have had a difficult time post-surgery, like me with a wound breakdown, still feel good about having a reduction. Breast reduction is the surgery that has the happiest results, according to research into cosmetic surgery.

I hope this book has helped you to decide whether a breast reduction is right for you and that if you do go ahead and have surgery, you know what to expect.

May your breasts be healthy. May you be happy. And may life be good.

Ayesha Hilton

PS Don't forget to claim your free bonus gifts to help you on your breast reduction journey. You will go on my mailing list, and I will share great information with you about all things breast reduction.

To get your free bonus gifts click the button or go to:
www.ayeshahilton.com/brsbonus

Glossary of Breast Reduction Terms

Areola Complex: The nipple and surrounding areola

Areola: Pigmented skin surrounding the nipple

Excision: To remove the skin

General Anesthesia: Drugs and/or gases used during an operation to relieve pain and alter consciousness

Breast Pedicle: An areola complex cut from the breast but attached by a cord of tissue to a part of the breast

Breast Reduction: Also known as reduction mammaplasty, the surgical removal of breast tissue to reduce the size of breasts

Free Nipple Graft (FNG): An areola complex that is cut completely free from any breast tissues

General anesthesia: Drugs and/or gases used during an operation to relieve pain and alter consciousness

Hematoma: Blood pooling beneath the skin

Incision: A surgical cut

Intravenous sedation: Sedatives administered by injection into a vein to help you relax

Liposuction: Also called lipoplasty or suction lipectomy, a procedure that vacuums out fat from beneath the skin's surface to reduce fullness

Local Anesthesia: A drug injected directly to the site of an incision during an operation to relieve pain

Mammogram: An x-ray image of the breast

Mastopexy: Surgery to lift the breasts

MRI (Magnetic Resonance Imaging): A painless test to view tissue, similar to an x-ray

Reduction mammoplasty: breast reduction, a surgical procedure that removes excess breast tissue to reshape the breast

Sutures: Stitches used by surgeons to hold skin and tissue together

About the Author:
Ayesha Hilton

Ayesha Hilton is an Amazon bestselling author, non-fiction book coach, avid learner, and spiritual adventurer.

As a young girl growing up in Melbourne, Australia, Ayesha dreamed of one day being a published author. She studied communications and professional writing at university and life got busy.

Life got busy, two kids were born, and she had almost forgotten her writing dream when she had an opportunity to co-write a book with her then farmer husband, Nick Shady, on farm succession planning. Their book, Who Gets the Farm? was a great success and has helped many farming families start talking about farm succession planning.

Since then, Ayesha has been a contributing author in a number of books, as well as writing several more of her own. She has created a range of journals and coloring books as well.

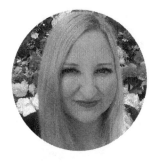

165

Connect with Ayesha

Ayesha Hilton Website

www.ayeshahilton.com

Facebook

www.ayeshahilton.com/facebook

LinkedIn

www.ayeshahilton.com/linkedin

Twitter

www.ayeshahilton.com/twitter

Instagram

www.ayeshahilton.com/instragram

Pinterest

www.ayeshahilton.com/pinterest

Acknowledgements

I would not have thought of writing this book if it weren't for the many women that reached out to me personally after they read my blog post about why I was going to have breast reduction.

I was surprised by the number of women who were considering having a breast reduction and were interested in my experience. I was equally surprised by how many women in my wider-circle of friends and acquaintances had already had breast reduction surgery.

It seemed so natural to document my experience and harness the shared experience of those who'd already been "under the knife" to collectively answer the many questions that women considering a reduction were asking.

With humility and appreciation, I wish to acknowledge those that have generously shared their knowledge, experience and support, and have had a direct impact on the writing of this book:

- To my then husband, Nick Shady (and his parents Bill and Yvonne Shady), who cared for our two children for the two weeks I was away having my breast reduction and post-op recovery – he did an amazing job and baked lots of cakes!

- My amazing friend of more than 20 years, AJ, who cared for me while I was recovering. You made my recovery more like a holiday and you spoilt me with your culinary delights, thank you.

- My father, Shaun Flanagan (affectionately known as Grandpa in our house), who takes my son on adventures and reads to my daughter before bed.

167

- All the women who answered my survey questions (for confidentiality reasons, I will not name you all here) – thank you for your honesty and for bravely sharing your personal stories.

- My surgeon and nursing staff – I am so glad I chose to have my surgery with you, my boobs are great!

Thank you to my new love, SB. Your love has helped me regain my enthusiasm for finishing this book. Your hugs are exactly what I need when I am stressed, and I feel so safe in your arms. I am excited for the next chapter in our lives together.

And finally, thank you dear reader, for taking the time out of your busy schedule to read my lovingly written book. I hope this book helps you decide whether a breast reduction is right for you. If you do choose to have a reduction, I hope this book gives you a good understanding of the process and the recovery.

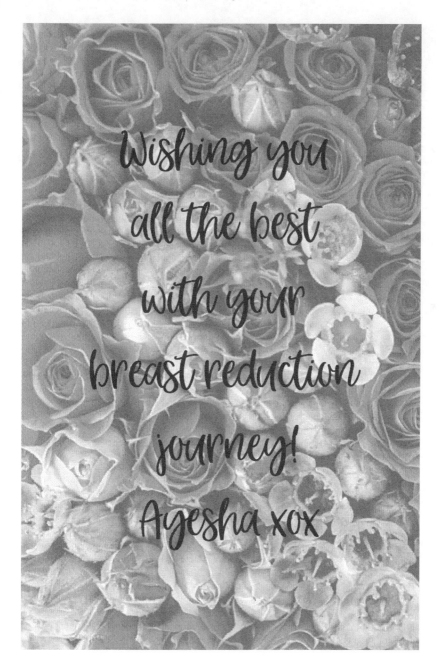

Wishing you all the best with your breast reduction journey! Ayesha xox

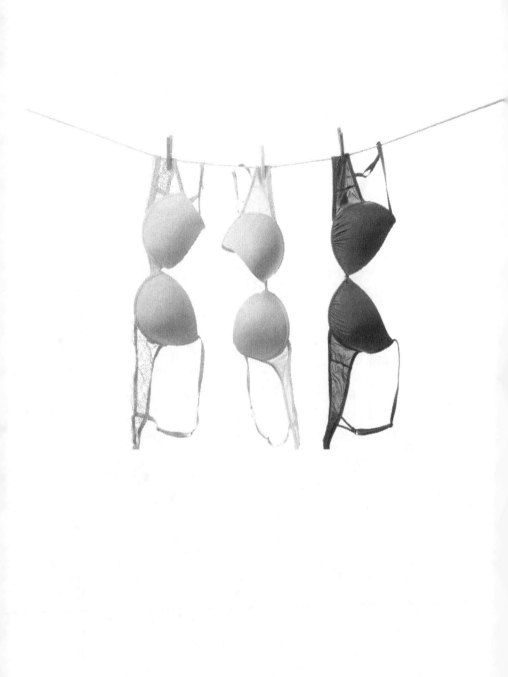

Made in the USA
Columbia, SC
19 September 2024

42599661R00100